Honey! I Shrunk the Tumor

Turning Wait Times Into Healing Times

Dea Cappelli

BALBOA.
PRESS

A DIVISION OF HAY HOUSE

Balboa Press books may be ordered through booksellers or by contacting:

Balboa Press
A Division of Hay House
1663 Liberty Drive
Bloomington, IN 47403
www.balboapress.com
1 (877) 407-4847

Because of the dynamic nature of the Internet, any web addresses or links contained in this book may have changed since publication and may no longer be valid. The views expressed in this work are solely those of the author and do not necessarily reflect the views of the publisher, and the publisher hereby disclaims any responsibility for them.

The author of this book does not dispense medical advice or prescribe the use of any technique as a form of treatment for physical, emotional, or medical problems without the advice of a physician, either directly or indirectly. The intent of the author is only to offer information of a general nature to help you in your quest for emotional and spiritual well-being. In the event you use any of the information in this book for yourself, which is your constitutional right, the author and the publisher assume no responsibility for your actions.

Any people depicted in stock imagery provided by Thinkstock are models, and such images are being used for illustrative purposes only. Certain stock imagery © Thinkstock.

Print information available on the last page.

ISBN: 978-1-5043-4356-5 (sc)
ISBN: 978-1-5043-4357-2 (e)

Balboa Press rev. date: 01/13/2016

Contents

In Remembrance of

Jo, dearest friend and aunt

Wonderful, whacky and glorious friends gone far too soon:

Inge, Suzanne, Gloria, Hilda, Yvonne, Roseanne, Evelyn, Betty

and darling Grandma, *mia Nonna*, who left so long ago

THE GUEST HOUSE

This being human is a guest house.
Every morning a new arrival.

A joy, a depression, a meanness,
some momentary awareness comes
as an unexpected visitor.

Welcome and entertain them all!
Even if they're a crowd of sorrows,
who violently sweep your house
empty of its furniture,
still, treat each guest honorably.
He may be clearing you out
for some new delight.

The dark thought, the shame, the malice,
meet them at the door laughing,
and invite them in.

Be grateful for whatever comes,
because each has been sent
as a guide from beyond.

Rumi
13th century Persian poet and mystic

This poem served as one of my guiding inspirations for my journey through the breast cancer.

Preface

Journal entry:
January 11, 2012
Writing on the eve of my fifth anniversary mammogram. Tomorrow I will be tested for the last time, or so I believe. I shall be declared "cancer-free".

Encouraged by my dear friend, Peter, to write this, I am reminded that over our lifetimes, we have several opportunities to check out. I was told, by a remarkable psychic, that I will look back at 90 years old, and realize that I have had three distinct lifetimes. And so, I recall the three chances I have had to leave this time around.

The first opportunity, when I was ten was later diagnosed with possible hepatitis. I was unable to maintain consciousness and kept "soaring to the stars". The doctor prepared my parents for my possible departure and many prayers were offered. Another psychic told me that I was turned back from heaven at that time, admonished since I still had a job to do.

My second chance also involved a loss of consciousness. Eighteen years ago, while in my forties, I was given a permanent pacemaker as I had lost consciousness five times in one afternoon. After I flat-lined in the ER, I sent the staff scurrying. I did have a premonition on that one, and again, I still had unfinished work to do. I had three children to educate and see married with children of their own.

I knew therefore, with my diagnosis of breast cancer, my third chance, that I would choose to stay. And so I put energy, research and practice into finding a way to let me remain here on earth so that I could help others facing the terrifying diagnosis of cancer and offer them hope and information to encourage and inspire them to lead a better, more beautiful life.

So who am I and upon what authority do I present these findings? I am your sister, a peace-loving teenager of the Beatles-era who grew up with a strong desire to be of service and make the world a better, safer place for all. Now, as grandmother to nine super kids and considering the state of world affairs politically and environmentally, that desire for peace is of even greater concern.

And so, heartened and strengthened by my life's experiences, and realizing that by tuning in holistically to what my "gut" felt was right, I embarked on my mission to shrink my breast cancer tumor. I share these *Reader's Digest-type* snippets of suggestions and scientific studies that will help you devise a unique plan that is right for you. You will find conventional treatments interspersed with new and old, proven alternative choices for you to explore further.

Like you, I have met many stresses and challenges throughout this lifetime: in personal relationships, health and finances. Some were emotional and tangible; others were environmental and imperceptible.

Besides my most important accomplishment – birthing and raising three wonderful children — I pursued careers as teacher of patients at a psychiatric hospital, then publisher of the *Canada Heirloom Series* and *Visual Convergence* magazine. Among various other endeavors, I worked as job developer for persons with disabilities and resume writer.

Along the way, I learned to tune into that which was unseen. Seeking to quiet my fears and doubts, I studied astrology, sought out psychics and looked for answers outside of myself. For many years I explored esoteric studies and meditation with a group of like-minded friends. I increasingly began to trust and rely on intuition and seek spiritual guidance from my higher power. I found that trying to remain in the moment presented opportunities to fine-tune the stirrings of my soul that I can only describe as knowing what is not evident through the senses. "Be still and know that I am God" became my mantra.

What is that knowing? Reaching into the innermost depths of being, it is a guidance that never fails. It can eliminate doubt, fear and anxiety. It is that still, small voice. Many times, this led to my overriding the advice of conventional medicine. When told my first baby, born seven weeks early, had suffered a brain injury trauma, I knew in my heart that the injury was marginal and that with determined effort he would overcome and thrive. And he did!

When a leading obstetrician suggested, due to my past history of two triple-high-risk pregnancies and a pending marital separation, that I abort my third unexpected pregnancy, I rejected his advice intuitively. As a result I am blessed with a beautiful daughter – my baby and light of my life. I simply *knew* all would work out well.

As a former teacher and publisher I find myself compelled to seek out and share information that I have uncovered. I truly feel I have been blessed and privileged and this is my opus of gratitude for the gifts that life presents every day: gifts of appreciation for nature in all its diverse forms and for life-affirming interpersonal relationships.

Part of the Earth community, we are all in this together; your journey is my journey. Come along with me; perhaps I will show you a way that you have not considered before.

Introduction

For many, the most distressing aspect of their journey through breast cancer is the waiting: for action, be it diagnosis, biopsy results, or a plan of treatment. Taking the position of one who waits is feeling powerless. There is nothing one can do to hasten the wheels of the powers that be. The only alleviating factor for me during my passage was the input of friends, all of whom knew of someone who had been through the demanding cancer labyrinth and who had survived and even thrived. Their stories were welcomed and inspiring and hopeful. Often, I was presented with reading material that served the intended purpose – to ease anxiety. One story was about a woman who actually made her tumor disappear!

Believing, as I do, that everything happens for a reason, I decided to use the infuriating "wait time" to my advantage. I would experiment with the various theories and treatments I was being exposed to and, if they were successful, I would share the teachings with others on a similar journey. My wait time would become my healing time.

There are those who claim to have had 100% remission of their breast cancer through alternative methods. This is not my claim. I urge you to try some self-healing for the effects of mitigating symptoms, maintaining positive thinking and increase well-being. The feeling of achieving some level of control can be a deliberate support during a difficult time. The information contained in this little book is for educational purposes and is provided as general information for you to use as you feel comfortable. It is not a scholarly treatise, after all, just a *Digest* of the research that is currently being done – a menu of options to choose from. This is an easy reference for you to pause and consider holistic options that best suit your lifestyle. Perhaps too, there is a gentle push to consider lifestyle changes that had not crossed your mind.

Some of these techniques may become lifelong habits and add to your quality of life. Your positive mental attitude will also have a calming effect on your loved ones who are also expressing frustrations, fear and delay. Dietary changes, proven to be cancer-preventing will assure optimal health and anti-aging – and who doesn't want that? Exercise will give added and necessary energy and strength. Both are prescribed for prevention of recurrence. Deep breathing and meditation will get you through so many of life's complications and rough spots and give every day an added dimension of inner peace and well-being.

I offer these findings with hope that you, too, my fellow traveler, may find, at the least, comfort and, at best, some reversal of this DIS-ease that has taken residence in your perfect body.

Chapter 1

Turning Wait Times into Healing Times

Delays, delays...

Journal entry:

November 2, 2006

> *Had lunch with Sheran... She says I mention "going" a lot. I must admit I think quite often of leaving this life.*

Although I discovered the unusual lump in October through self-exam, I did not see my family doctor until early December and casually mentioned the bump in my right breast. I've known my doctor since we were youngsters and recognized the look of concern on his face.

December 8

> *None of the psychics at the Christmas party mentioned the lump in my breast. Dr. Z is concerned. I have a mammogram booked. How will I cope with loss of income?*

I should be able to do it, but do I want to? Have I finished what I came to do? I want to stay to complete my promise to take care of Mom. I want to stay to mentor Alexandrea and help with Matty's care and Rachel, Ryan and Kyle. I want to see my grandchildren grow and thrive. I want to see Jamie's children some day.

"There's always something!" as Gilda Radner used to say.

I must be depressed, but don't feel it.

In the meantime, it's work, work, work!!!

Dec. 10

At lunch with Sheran, she says, the decision to go is a decision. She gave me Adam's book, Adam Dreamhealer.

I meditated this a.m. I have decided to stay and fight. Going at this stage is selfishness, laziness and copping out.

I have a plan:
- *Daily meditations to get rid of lump*
- *Exercise 3X week instead of TV*
- *More involvement with grandchildren*
- *As I prepare for income taxes, I will get finance paperwork in order*
- *I will purge and de-clutter and excise materialism*
- *I will sell off on eBay and Kijiji*
- *I ask dear departed Dad and Jo to help with this decision. I know from both and from Doris that to help and care for the dying is an honour and know*

that when time comes, my family will be there for me – but that time is not for a long time.

Live life fully now. This can be done without money:
Enjoy the outdoors, hiking, gardening and vacationing.
Enjoy your talents: painting, sculpting, cooking (yes you do have some modest ability!), decorating, dancing (where and with whom?)
Entertaining, writing....
So the next few weeks address a lot of issues:

- *Pacemaker clinic*
- *Bone density test*
- *Blood tests, mammogram*
- *New pacemaker*
- *Eye exam*
- *Sleepover for Rachel, Sydney and Lauren*

On Monday, I called the breast screening clinic and asked for a cancellation appointment for quicker results.

Somehow, I did manage to get an appointment for mid-December. They were over-booked and I waited all day to be seen as the last appointment. After looking at my X-ray, the nurse was very empathetic and suggested I return with a friend for the radiologist's report and subsequent biopsy. Because we were about to begin Christmas break, this would be done in the New Year.

Dec. 21

Winter solstice and new moon. A new beginning for sure
Today is my mammogram date. I will soon have assurance that
everything is OK. In the meantime I have made contingency
plans which I shall carry out either way:
- *be kind good and loving to Dea, No more deprivations,*
  only the best
- *Get rid of clutter*
- *Continue positive direction in relationship with Mom*
- *Devote more time to health, exercise diet,*
  meditation; have FUN
- *What is fun? Movies, museums, games, get kids to*
  play with me. We had such fun at cottage.
- *Friends to enlist: Monica, Leytha, Sylvia, Pam, Judy,*
  Sheran, Ginny, Christine, Helen, Gloria

And some male energy:
Jason, Jamie, Ilo, Chris, Adam, Gil, Charlie and Tom.
That's quite a support team!
- *Plan a sunshine holiday*
- *Knit, write letters, read*
- *Organize photographs*
- *I will pay minimum credit balances to have a safety*
  net in case!
- *6:15; time for a nap. I am calm and optimistic*

And so we have Christmas this week-end. It will be good!

Not wanting to put a damper on holiday cheer, I kept the secret to myself and told only my closest friend, Monica, on a blustery winter's walk, just before New Year's.

After the Christmas holiday closure, I arrived at the clinic ready to have the lump biopsied. The attending physician for the day, seeing my history chart, asked if I had taken aspirin. I do take a daily baby aspirin and replied affirmatively. She then refused to do the biopsy stating I had to be aspirin-free for a week. Of course, if I had been told two weeks ago about this potential problem, I would have remained aspirin-free. As it was, I had to return in another week. Another delay!

I returned the next week with Monica, a loving friend who was my constant source of support through the whole ordeal, and, although we were booked for 9:30, we waited all morning amongst a large crowd of women awaiting their turns for mammograms. Mid-afternoon, I insisted Monica go back to her work one hour out of town. By the time it was my turn for biopsy, there was little time before clinic closing for the anaesthetic to take hold. Because the ultrasound machine was overbooked, I was told my breast would be held steady for the procedure in the mammogram machine which "would only take about 10 minutes".

Ten minutes in the mammogram machine!!! Oh, no, not me. I insisted that since I had waited all day I would get the more humane treatment. Since the anaesthetic had not fully taken hold, I felt the needle stab and to say it stung is an understatement! But it was done.

Armed with care instructions, I would await the results for a week or so.

Test Results Time

When I visited my GP for the test results, my doctor was unable to download them as the laboratory's website server was down. Sweet Dr. Z. called the lab directly and after some delay was given the verbal report. It was, as we suspected, Cancer: a stage 2, hormone receptive, 2 cm. malignant tumour.

An appointment with a surgeon was arranged immediately. Dr. Z. assured me I would be OK. He knows my determined nature and I appreciated his confidence in the outcome. My referred surgeon was "the best in the city."

And so my self-healing began...

> I opted for lumpectomy (removal of the lump) and sentinel node lymphectomy (removal and examination of the first two lymph nodes) with radiation treatments to follow. This is the prescribed protocol for stage 2 based on the size of the lump.

> It was by accident that I discovered that my lump had shrunk during the five weeks from biopsy to surgery.

> After the surgery, at the follow-up visit to the surgeon, I asked for a copy of the post-operative biopsy report. The tumor was reported 1.5 cm at its largest radius. I thought at first it was an error in the initial sizing. A few days later, in the middle of the night, -- a time when truth often reveals itself -- I woke up startled by the thought that my tumor had indeed shrunk by almost 25%!

> How had I done that?

Fourteen years earlier I had been given another opportunity to heal myself. Perhaps then if I had chosen to write about it, I would not have had to experience a second chance to heal and share. (Remember, I believe everything that happens and the people we meet in our lives are there for a purpose!)

I had been experiencing bouts of arrhythmias and ignored them until one day, due to business financial problems and the stresses of a relationship breakup, I blacked out five times in one day. Unable to stay conscious and even flat-lining in a hospital ER, I was immediately given a temporary heart pacemaker once a brain tumour was ruled out. A permanent pacemaker was implanted two days later. (My diagnosis was Sick Sinus Syndrome, which was exceptionally rare for a person in her forties — most patients are in their '80s.) During clinic visits following, it was determined that I was 87% dependent on the pacemaker to keep my heartbeat going.

After a year or so, I decided to visit a naturopathic doctor and he, Dr. McKenzie, put me on a holistic regime which I credit for reducing my dependency on the pacemaker to less than 1% still today. Some of his recommendations (especially the visualizations specific for heart-healing) are the same ones I include in this book for my breast cancer "healing".

Ironically, it was my pacemaker replacement, due at the very same time as a course of radiation was ordered, that led to even further delay for treatment – each separate hospital clinic wanted the procedure to be done first by the other.

As luck would have it, in the course of researching Pathfinders Canadian Tributes, I met and had lunch with Dr. Wilfred G.

"Bill" Bigelow, OC FRSC (June 18, 1913 – March 27, 2005) a Canadian heart surgeon known for his role in developing the artificial pacemaker and the use of hypothermia in open heart surgery. I had the opportunity to personally thank him for that lifesaver and also his work on Heparin. A truly remarkable and beautiful man!

Chapter 2

Arm Yourself

My experience was very different from many that I have read about. In the grand scheme of things I do not count it as one of my life's most devastating experiences and there have been a few of those! Intuitively, I knew I would overcome. I was unable to continue reading Doctor Marla Shapiro's excellent book, *Life in the Balance*, because I found it so gut-wrenching and my experience was not close to being as horrendous. I did find that book very interesting after the fact, but it was upsetting before surgery and I was determined to remain as clear-headed and as positive as possible. As my journey was less traumatic than that of many, I have tried to make this book light and informative, an everyday reference that anyone can relate to and can use to incorporate suggestions into everyday life.

While considered rare, male breast cancer represents about 1% of all breast cancers. The male breast has less tissue mass than the female and the tumor spreads rapidly and infiltrates the underlying muscle and overlapping skin. Ulceration though the skin is common. Tumor spread throughout the surrounding tissues and lymph nodes is similar to that of the female. The treatments, regimens, prognosis and recovery are the same for both sexes.

You will hear that every case is unique and each treatment plan tailor-made. With this in mind, I urge you to learn as much as you can about the options available before and after surgery.

In this chapter, I have summarized what you need to know immediately after diagnosis while preparing for treatment and recovery. Later, in Chapter 3, some strategies to work directly on shrinking the tumor and minimizing effects of treatments are uncovered. Then, in Chapter 5, preventive strategies with life-style changes and adaptations will be presented.

Wait Times

The good news is that the delays give you time to condition your body and strengthen your immune system in order to promote quicker, easier healing. Like preparing for a marathon, (something I have not ever remotely even considered!), conditioning reduces shock and that lessens side effects of surgery and radiation. I very stringently followed all skin care advice so that pacemaker surgery three weeks later, in spite of the implant being on the same side as the radiation therapy, there was no problem with healing. As a matter of fact, the surgeon remarked, "You have beautiful skin. You will heal well." And I did!

There is a lot going on behind the scenes that you may not be aware of. My oncology specialists conferred with the cardiac specialist about the best course of action when there was concern over which should be performed first: radiation or pacemaker replacement surgery. Earlier, when I requested both surgeries be performed at the same time, the two surgery specialists conferred and determined that this was not the best course of action. But they did respectfully consider and discuss my request.

When I questioned my radiologist about wait times following a negative newspaper report, he assured me there is a method in place to assure that those most in need receive treatment first.

One thing that I did not know – but wish I had found out earlier – was that my type of tumor grows slowly and the lack of quick medical response is not crucial to a positive outcome in the early stages of breast cancer. I was amazed to learn that my 2 cm tumor would probably have been growing for 10 years before it was detected. I did not realize, when I first observed a large blue vein just above the pacemaker, that more prominent veins in one breast can be an early sign of breast cancer. That was 14 years before diagnosis. (At that time, I questioned the cardiac surgeon and he attributed it to a blood clot. I wonder if the two are related.)

My advice: try to stay positive (you will hear that a lot!) and remember that each experience is different.

Prepare for your oncology consult with a small notebook and written questions

- Carry a notepad and pen at all times and start an information file.
- Collect business cards from all appointments.
- Schedule an appointment with your doctor and ask questions that YOU want answers to.
- If possible, audibly record every medical visit. You can listen later to clarify until you really "get it".
- Ask an attentive friend, someone who is willing to speak up for you and take notes, to accompany you.
- Review your questions ahead of time.

- Questions you may ask:
    - What does hormone receptive mean?
    - What is Her2 receptive?
    - What is Staging? *
    - What is Typing?
    - What is Grading?
    - What about Radiation?
    - What about chemotherapy?

*for staging info:
http://www.nccn.org/patients/patient_gls/_english/_breast/4_stages.asp
Click on download for the pdf booklet. It gives chapters with all the info you need.

Here are some questions you can ask your oncologist about your risk of recurrence:

- How often does this cancer reoccur in healthy women?
- What are the symptoms of a recurrence?
- When do I schedule an appointment regarding symptoms?
- What are my risk factors regarding recurrence?
- Are there lifestyle changes I can make or medical treatment plans we could discuss that might prevent recurrence?

With the growing volume of alternative, holistic choices out there, I really feel the need to encourage you to listen to your body and your gut-feelings, especially on the matter of choosing the best plan of action. Each one of us is unique and only you know you. Do not make your decision in a rush! Breast cancer is usually not an emergency. Take time to weigh your options.

Remember:
"All scientific work is incomplete and liable to be upset or modified by advancing knowledge. That does not confer on us a freedom to ignore the knowledge we already have or postpone the action that it appears to demand at a given time."

Bradford Hill
Management of Imperfect Evidence, 1965

From Dr. Joseph Mercola's article, " Top Ten Ways the American Health Care System Fails":
"From time to time, medical experts reverse course on certain practices and procedures when science dictates a change in the standard of care. One classic example of a "reversal" is when hormone therapy for menopausal women came to a screeching halt when so many women developed blood clots, stroke, and breast and uterine cancers."

<http://articles.mercola.com/sites/articles/archive/2014/03/15/bad-american-health-care-system.aspx?e_cid=20140315Z1_DNL_art_1&utm_source=dnl&utm_medium=email&utm_content=art1&utm_campaign=20140315Z1&et_cid=DM40734&et_rid=457435104>

Treatments

Radiation therapy uses beams of intense energy to kill cancer cells most often from X-rays. It is recommended following lumpectomy to eliminate any microscopic cancer cells in the remaining breast tissue. Eighty percent to 90 percent of women treated with modern surgery and radiation therapy techniques have excellent or good cosmetic results: that is, little or no change in treated breast in size, shape, texture or appearance compared with what it was like before treatment. Years of clinical study have proven that this **breast conservation therapy** offers the same cure rate as mastectomy (having the entire breast removed).

There are several studies in which older patients with small tumors have had a local relapse when treated with lumpectomy and hormonal therapy **without radiation**. This issue should be discussed in detail with your doctor, as there is still uncertainty about long-term results with this approach or about which individuals will do best without radiation therapy.

Accelerated hypo-fractionated whole breast irradiation, an intense three week course of radiation therapy, is just as effective as the standard five week regimen for women with early-stage breast cancer says a team of researchers led by Hamilton, Ontario, McMaster University oncology professor Dr. Timothy J. Whelan. This was the schedule to which I was lucky to be assigned. In an early-stage trial, additional radiation to the lymph nodes only prevented the spread of cancer by an estimated 30% disease-free survival rate.

Risks of Radiation Therapy

By Mayo Clinic staff

Side effects of radiation therapy greatly depend on which part of your body is being exposed to radiation and how much radiation is used. You may experience no side effects, or you may experience several. Most side effects are temporary, can be controlled and generally disappear over time once treatment has ended.

Some side effects may develop later. For example, in rare circumstances a new cancer (second primary cancer) that's different from the first one treated with radiation may develop years later. Ask your doctor about potential side effects, both short and long term, which may occur after your treatment.

Mayo Clinic Staff 17 June 2015 <http://www.mayoclinic.org/tests-procedures/radiation-therapy-for-breast-cancer/basics/why-its-done/prc-20013445>

Sentinel node biopsy is a surgical procedure used to determine if cancer has spread beyond a primary tumor into your lymphatic system. Sentinel node biopsy is used most commonly in evaluating breast cancer and melanoma.

The **lymphatic system** is a series of vessels throughout the body that drain fluid from tissues. Bacteria and other microbes are picked up in the lymphatic fluid and trapped inside lymph nodes, where they can be attacked and destroyed by white blood cells. The sentinel nodes are the first few lymph nodes into which a tumor drains. Sentinel node biopsy involves injecting a tracer material that helps the surgeon locate the sentinel nodes during surgery. The sentinel nodes are removed and analyzed in a laboratory. If the sentinel nodes are free of cancer, then cancer isn't likely to have spread and removing additional lymph nodes is unnecessary.

If, after sentinel node biopsy, evaluation of the sentinel nodes reveals cancer, then you'll likely need additional lymph nodes removed for your doctor to determine how far the cancer has spread.

New research suggests that up to 20% of patients could be spared aggressive node surgery and possible troubling side effects. However, this typically applies to women with relatively early disease, with spread to no more than two nodes.

Brachytherapy is a form of radiotherapy that involves implanting radioactive "seeds" inside or near a malignant tumor. The seeds work like tiny time-release capsules blasting the affected area directly rather than blasting through layers of healthy tissues in standard radiation therapy. It takes hours not weeks, has little impact on healthy cells and can be more effective at killing cancer for good.

Chemotherapy for Breast Cancer

By Mayo Clinic staff

Chemotherapy for breast cancer uses powerful drugs to target and destroy fast-growing cancer cells. Chemotherapy is frequently used along with other treatments, such as surgery. But chemotherapy for breast cancer also may be used as the primary treatment, when surgery is not an option.

Breast cancer chemotherapy drugs may be used individually or in combination to increase the effectiveness of the treatment. Chemotherapy can help you live longer and reduce your chances of having the cancer come back (recur), but also carries a risk of side effects: some temporary and mild, others more serious or permanent. Your doctor can help you decide whether chemotherapy for breast cancer is a good choice for you. Be sure to discuss long-term effects!

Mayo Clinic, 17 June 2015: <http://www.mayoclinic.org/tests-procedures/chemotherapy-for-breast-cancer/basics/definition/prc-20013035>

It has been suggested that Vitamin C may decrease the effectiveness of cancer-fighting drugs. It is worth a discussion with your doctors to find out if this affects your situation.

Now consider this.

From © 2009 Dr. James Howenstine

"All Rights Reserved: Anyone reading this article has my permission to copy or publish this information. Hopefully, some individuals will be made aware that there are safe effective alternatives to chemotherapy and radiation in the treatment of malignancies."

The package inserts for chemotherapy drugs admit that taking a course of chemotherapy drugs can increase your risk of subsequently developing a new cancer by about 10%. The National Institute for Occupational Safety and Health (NIOSH) warns that the powerful drugs used in chemotherapy can cause cancer in employees who handle them (nurses, pharmacists, cleaning personnel). If continued too long these drugs are fatal. The damage to white blood cell, killer lymphocyte and red blood cell production makes the patient vulnerable to overwhelming infection which is the cause of death in many patients on chemotherapy and radiation. It never made sense to me why administering toxic substances that cause major side effects could possibly heal a serious illness like a malignancy.

> Dr. William Campbell Douglass II, MD: "To understand the utter hypocrisy of chemotherapy, consider the following: The McGill Cancer Center in Canada, one of the largest and most prestigious cancer treatment centers in the world, did a study of oncologists to determine how they would respond to a diagnosis of cancer. On the confidential questionnaire, 58 out of 64 doctors said that all chemotherapy programs were unacceptable to them and their family.

Furthermore:

Chemotherapy shows very little success with common solid tumors that occur in the colon, lung and breasts, as documented over the past decade, yet somehow "chemo" is still recommended to attempt to stave off tumors and malignant growths in these areas of the body.

Learn more: http://www.naturalnews.com/036054_chemotherapy physicians_toxicity.html##ixzz2vafZ2zXX

Take note:

Resveratrol, a potent antioxidant found in a number of plants, including red grape skins, pomegranate, raw cacao, peanuts, and berries like raspberries and mulberries, is known to have a number of beneficial health effects. It also shows promise both as a natural substance that can help you overcome resistance to chemotherapy drugs — and increase the effectiveness of radiation therapy.

Cancer immunotherapy, which uses the body's immune system to help fight cancer cells, has been named by *Science Magazine* as the "breakthrough" scientific achievement of 2013. The magazine's editors say that even though the treatment is still in its early stages, **immunotherapy** is shifting the way cancer researchers are thinking about how to treat the disease, from targeting the tumor to enlisting the immune system to destroy the tumor.

The Canadian Cancer Society funds a number of promising research projects focusing on **immunotherapy** using T cells and ultimately make immunotherapies more effective.

Read more: <http://www.cancer.ca/en/about-us/news/national/ 2014/boosting-the-immune-system-to-defend-the-body-against-cancer/?region=on&utm_medium=SponsoredBulletin&utm_ content=Immunotherapy&utm_campaign=DONATIONS_ON_ BoomerTest_2014#ixzz2vgXgYy00>

In chapter 3, Adam Dreamhealer's self-healing tips on rallying your T cells into cancer-fighting action are described further.

There are some possible concerns to be aware of following breast cancer treatment.

Lymphedema (lymphatic fluid buildup) is the most common health concern related to surgical procedures. This swelling can occur in the arm or armpit area and may begin days or even years after surgery for breast cancer. Report any swelling or tightness in your arm to your doctor immediately!

If you had a mastectomy, you may also experience what doctors call **"phantom pain,"** or pain that seems to be coming from your missing breast. This should resolve over time. Talk to your doctor if the pain becomes particularly bothersome. Pain-relief medicine may be recommended.

Patients who undergo radiation can experience **skin irritation** at the radiation site. This irritation will fade away slowly and typically be gone within 12 months.

Radiation can also worsen **lymphedema** which can be caused by surgery to treat breast cancer. Radiation to the chest area can also cause **radiation pneumonitis**. This is a rare condition and can cause a dry cough and trouble breathing. Talk to your doctor immediately if you experience these symptoms.

<http://breastcancer.about.com/od/whattoexpect/tp/Staying-Healthy-At-Work-During-Breast-Cancer-Treatment.htm>

Adjuvant Therapy

After surgery and perhaps chemotherapy and radiation, you may be placed on **adjuvant therapy** (treatment that is given in addition to the primary, main or initial treatment) to help prevent recurrence. If you are premenopausal, your therapy may be **tamoxifen**; if you are postmenopausal, it may be one of the newer aromatase inhibitors such as **Arimidex**. (Aromatase inhibitors stop the production of estrogen in postmenopausal women.) It is advised to continue the adjuvant therapy up to five years. Studies on tamoxifen showed that women who used it for five years reduced breast cancer recurrence rate by 41 percent and mortality by 34% in patients with ER+ tumors compared with placebo.

In a study published in *The Lancet,* July 2015, aromatase inhibitors were found to reduce death rates by 40 per cent within 10 years of starting treatment.

Sleep environment may affect Tamoxifen's effectiveness so taking it one hour before bedtime you can take advantage of the body's natural increase in melatonin production at night.

A far less toxic alternative to Tamoxifen is raloxifene (**Evista**) used to treat osteoporosis. In one study women who took Evista had 55% reduction risk of developing invasive ER-positive breast cancer than those taking a placebo. However, Evista's breast cancer prevention benefits were less than that of tamoxifen.

April 17

> *Sylvia accompanied me to meet Oncologist. The doctor was thorough in her explanation of biopsy report, options and examination. Suggested a colonoscopy.*
> *Decided for several reasons on Tamoxifen for 2.5 years then a switch to anastrozole. Cost differences were significant; side effects were considered.*
> *Syl and I had lunch at La Luna – just like old times*
> *Will start Tamoxifen tomorrow and exercise today!*

Arimidex can cause heart problems. And tamoxifen can cause uterine cancer. Since I have heart issues (sort of) and have had a hysterectomy, I chose Tamoxifen. (Plus, it's much less expensive for those not on a drug plan!)

April 21

> *So far no side effects from Tamoxifen. Cried a little when pharmacist told me of side effects. Hair loss perturbed me most. Got over it fast realizing I am a lucky one and my journey is a lot easier than that of so many.*

Sleeping better – waking at 6 instead of 3 and more dreams. On T since 5 days, no other changes to report. But – I had to nap yesterday, a rarity for me.

April 30

Almost 2 weeks of Tamoxifen and had a very energetic "up" weekend. I was bound to crash and I did!
But earlier in the day I visited radiologist at the Juravinski with Sylvia who took copious notes on everything he said! He was great and arranged for me to see him again tomorrow. So once again I was lucky. Syl took notes and listened for me (my poor listening skills have diminished even more). There is so much going on and my concentration can waiver so.

Easing the Pain

In a Korean study (2005) 30 breast cancer patients were given **progressive muscle realization therapy** (PMRT) and taught to use guided imagery during their six months of **chemotherapy**. Another 30 were treated with chemo alone. The first group experienced less nausea and vomiting and members were less anxious, depressed and irritable than those receiving chemo alone. Six months after treatment ended, the PMRT and guided imagery group was still experiencing a better quality of life than the group that did not receive training.

Music can help cancer patients ease their anxiety and improve their mood, pain, and quality of life. That's the conclusion of a study of nearly 2000 patients at Drexel University in Philadelphia. In addition, the researchers found listening to **music** brought about a considerable reduction in heart and respiratory rates, and blood pressure when patients listened to pre-recorded music or had sessions with trained music therapists.

Ear acupuncture helps control night sweats and hot flashes for women receiving breast cancer treatment. Patients reported over 35% reduction in symptoms.

Cancer patients should consider **exercise** to help overcome cancer-related fatigue (CRF). CRF not only weakens a patient physically, it also reduces mental ability. Experts recommend and several studies conclude that exercise can reduce fatigue and increase quality of life in patients undergoing cancer treatment. Source: <oawhealth.com>

Recently many researchers have been getting excited about **frankincense oil**. More and more evidence is growing that this natural oil may provide a powerful way to fight cancer. The active ingredients in the sacred frankincense oil were shown to activate an "immune cells attack" against cancer cells meaning that the frankincense oil was activating immune cells in the body and effectively supporting the body in attacking and destroying cancer cells.

The studies found that the most effective time to start using the frankincense oil as a treatment was before any other treatments began. My introduction to essential oils came years later and I was not able to implement this effective treatment.

Melatonin's Impressive Role in Fighting Cancer

Melatonin is a powerful breast cancer fighter: a potent anti-oxidant, it is five times more powerful than Vitamin C and twice that of Vitamin E.

Melatonin is a hormone your body produces at night, and one of its primary roles is to help you sleep. Melatonin may help protect against heart disease, diabetes, Alzheimer's and migraine headaches. Melatonin may also help with weight control and strengthening your immune system.

Published research has shown melatonin offers particularly strong protection against reproductive cancers. Cells throughout your body — even cancer cells — have melatonin receptors.

So when melatonin's production peaks during the night, cell division slows. When this hormone latches onto a breast cancer cell, it has been found to counteract estrogen's tendency to stimulate cell growth.

In fact, melatonin has a calming effect on several reproductive hormones, which may explain why it seems to protect against sex hormone-driven cancers, including ovarian, endometrial, breast, prostate and testicular cancers.

GreenMedInfo.com lists 20 studies demonstrating exactly how melatonin exerts its protective effects against breast cancer.

While causing cancer cells to self-destruct, melatonin also boosts your production of immune-optimizing substances such as interleukin-2, which helps identify and attack the mutated cells that lead to malignant cancer.

The greatest area of melatonin research to date is related to breast cancer. Some of the more impressive studies include the following:

Exposing Yourself to Light at Night Shuts Down Your Melatonin and Raises Your Cancer Risk <http://articles.mercola.com/sites/ articles/archive/2013/03/19/melatonin-benefits.aspx>

- The journal *Epidemiology* (January 2001) reported increased breast cancer risk among women who work predominantly night shifts
- Women who live in neighborhoods with large amounts of nighttime illumination are 30-50% more likely to get breast cancer than those who live in areas where nocturnal darkness prevails, according to an Israeli study. (*Cancer Causes Control,* December 2010).
- From participants in the Nurses' Health Study, it was found that nurses who work nights had 36 percent higher rates of breast cancer (*Journal National Cancer Institute, August 2001*)
- Blind women, whose eyes cannot detect light and so have robust production of melatonin, have lower-than-average breast cancer rates (*Epidemiology,* September 1998)

When you turn on a light at night, your biological clock instructs your pineal gland to immediately stop producing melatonin; sleeping in complete darkness is important for healthful melatonin production.

➢ Forego bright overhead lights in the evening. Instead, use task lights; use a low red bulb night light in your bedroom and bathroom to block out the blue-wavelength light during sleep.

New research suggests that an increase in magnetic field strength in a woman's bedroom is associated with a reduction in melatonin production. Animal experiments show that magnetic fields suppress melatonin production and accelerate the growth of breast tumors. Some studies indicate that very strong magnetic fields, such as those experienced by power line workers, may increase the risk of male breast cancer.

I tell all who will listen to wear a sleep mask at night for complete darkness. Once you try it you will never go without!

Foods and Herbs for Healing Cancer

Personally, I cannot stress enough the importance of increasing wholesome, organically grown foods into your lifestyle. There are many proven powerhouse cancer-fighters and they are all in the garden-variety and that is why organic is important – adding pesticides to the growing will have the opposite effect. You will find no animal products in the lists studied and mentioned here!

Natural News writer Derek Henry details them:

Sea Vegetables
Kelp, kombu, and nori are three of the more common sea vegetables with remarkable effects on cancer. They are one of the richest and most bioavailable sources of **iodine,** a substance lacking in the average diet that is implicated in many patients with breast and ovarian cancer. Iodine has potent anticancer properties and has been shown to cause cell death in breast and thyroid cancer cells.

They are also rich in calcium and potassium, as well as all minerals, which assist in promoting a very alkaline environment, which makes it very difficult for existing cancer to survive.

Algae

Chlorella and spirulina are two of the most potent algae and are proven cancer fighters. Due to their incredible detoxification action including binding to and eliminating heavy metals and immune-boosting properties by promoting production of healthy gut flora and fighting candida overgrowth, they are a valuable consideration in healing cancer.

Cruciferous Vegetables

Cruciferous vegetables like broccoli, cauliflower, Brussel sprouts and cabbage have been linked to lower cancer risks and have the ability to halt growth of cancer cells for tumors in the breast, lung, colon, liver, and cervix.

Broccoli has been repeatedly shown to be one of nature's most valuable health-promoting foods, capable of preventing a number of health issues, including hypertension, allergies, diabetes, osteoarthritis and cancer.

Recent tests on cells, tissues and mice show that a broccoli compound has also been shown to kill cancer stem cells, thereby slowing tumor growth. It appears that broccoli contains the necessary ingredients to switch ON genes that prevent cancer development, and switch OFF other ones that help it spread.

Research has shown that fresh broccoli sprouts contain 20 to 50 times the amount of chemo-protective compounds found in mature broccoli heads.

Medicinal Mushrooms

Medicinal mushrooms such as reishi and chaga have had a number of bioactive molecules, including anti-tumor agents, identified in their structure.

Studies show that long-term consumption of reishi prevents tumor growth by increasing the level of antioxidants in an individual's blood plasma while boosting the immunity of those suffering from advanced stage cancer.

Aloe Vera

A study in *International Immuno-pharmacology* showed that aloe vera has anti-tumor potential. Researchers found that aloe vera, available in health food stores, boosts immune system function and destroys cancer tumors.

Hemp

The **hemp** plant contains some of the most balanced and richest sources of oils on the planet, with an ideal ratio of 3:1 for omega 6 to omega 3. **Hemp seed oil** also contains 80% essential fatty acids (EFAs), the highest of any plant. Essential fatty acids are fundamental to immune function due to their antioxidants and anti-inflammatory fatty acids, which helps oxidize the cells and restores health at a cellular level. Since cancer cannot survive in a highly oxygenated environment, the superb EFA content in hemp makes it a great option for helping to healing cancer.

Turmeric

The Life Extension Foundation has conducted extensive research into the anti-cancer properties of turmeric and found that it targets 10 causative factors involved in cancer development, including DNA damage, chronic inflammation, and disruption of cell signaling pathways.

Hundreds of studies have also shown that **curcumin**, a substance in turmeric is a potent anti-cancer food that blocks cancer development in a number of unique ways.

Learn more:
<http://www.naturalnews.com/044443_healing_foods_cancer_immune_support.html>

And as previously mentioned, **turmeric** extract decreases inflammation and increases tumor suppression. Research in animals has shown turmeric makes cancer cells more susceptible to radiation therapy at the same time protecting normal cells against damage.

Bee Propolis

A substance that honey bees collect from tree buds, sap flows, or other botanical sources has powerful immune-modulating, anti-inflammatory properties. CAPE, one of the main active compounds of bee propolis, even when used in low doses, can prevent cellular mistakes in healthy cells and induce cell death in cancer cells. Thus it seems to have a double benefit of protecting healthy cells while killing cancer cells. (Chen et al 2003).

By using water-soluble **bee propolis**, researchers experimented on mice with breast tumors to show antioxidants can enhance the performance of both radiation and chemotherapy. This supports the work of Chen noted above, that CAPE can cause cell death, while protecting the DNA of healthy cells

My dear friend Monica gave me a dropper bottle of **bee propolis** with instructions from a Romanian physician–healer to use 10 drops on dry bread first thing every morning one-half hour before eating. I still use it now and again. Evidently there is no limit to the daily intake and no toxic or adverse side effects have been reported. (Providing you are not allergic to the substance, of course!)

*****

I have tried my best to include, at time of printing, the latest research, but this is not an exhaustive list. There are many other strategies that can be useful as well. One excellent resource is *Waking the Warrior Goddess: Dr. Christine Horner's Program to Protect Against and Fight Breast Cancer,* which contains research-proven all-natural approaches for protecting against and treating breast cancer.

Now we are ready to explore adjunct and alternative methods of mitigating symptoms and promoting self-healing through allopathic, naturopathic and holistic medicine.

Chapter 3

Stretch Yourself

The wound is the place where the light enters you.

Rumi

The popularity of Dr. Oz's TV program and Dr. Mercola's web–based presentations and the many published books and articles on the subject is a testament to the growing interest in holistic therapies. Many patients living with dis-ease desire to integrate mainstream medicine with some forms of alternative/complementary medicine in their revised lifestyles.

Modern research on most complementary/holistic therapies is relatively new and most of the studies are small. Remember, however, that they have been healing humans since the dawn of time. Many believe that, when combined with conventional medicine, complementary/holistic therapies offer a more integrated approach to healing. The American Cancer Society recommends that if holistic medicine is to be used at all, it should be used only in conjunction with conventional medicine and not as a replacement.

Personally, I have tried most of these described below and heartily recommend them all. Ideally, healing of the spirit, mind, emotions and body should be embraced for a lifetime of whole, healthy living.

Healing the Body

Many different healing modalities have been proven to be effective in relieving pain, anxiety and bothersome side effects of breast cancer treatments. All can benefit everyone's life no matter what ailment or discomfort that may be encountered. Here are some that I explored.

ywcaencore ™ offered by the YWCA Hamilton, Ontario, is a free post-breast cancer program customized to complement the medical treatment of breast cancer for women who have experienced mastectomy, lumpectomy or breast reconstruction. The program is based around gentle floor and pool exercises and relaxation techniques that are safe, fun and therapeutic. Healthy snacks, educational sessions with guests speakers, support from a network of friends and exercise therapy that can help you take control of your life are offered. I find myself channeling in to the good advice and inspirational energy encountered in the sessions many times when I need a kick-start to exercise. Yearly reunions are very informative and fun! Contact acollingwood@ ywcahamilton.org for more info. Every community should have an encore program!

Who has not tried or at least thought about trying yoga? **Yoga** is the ancient Indian practice for mind-body wellness. Western yoga can be a valuable addition to the process of healing and recovery, especially during and following treatments. Fatigue, pain, swelling, stiffness, stress, and depression have been shown time and again to be alleviated by yoga in one of its many forms.

In particular, I like restorative yoga, a gentle, non-competitive practice to restore and revitalize.

It has been shown that practitioners of yoga have lower levels of cortisol, the stress hormone which may contribute to cancer recurrence and earlier mortality among breast cancer survivors.

I found that yoga made me stronger and more flexible and more relaxed. I highly recommend that you search your community for customized classes for cancer patients and survivors.

Therapeutic massage, first described in China around 2500 years ago was used by Hippocrates to treat sprains. Researchers at University of Miami following breast cancer patients for 5 weeks found that women in the massage group reported feeling less depressed and angry and had more energy than those using muscle relaxation therapy.

Acupuncture is an ancient tradition that uses needles to stimulate the body's pressure points. An American study provides evidence that acupuncture can help ease hot flashes in women being treated with the anti-estrogen drug, **tamoxifen**. Acupuncture, researchers found, is free of side effects and has a side benefit for some women: an increased sex drive. In a trial comparing Effexor and acupuncture, both reduced night sweats and hot flashes and depression to a similar degree. But weeks after treatment ended, the Effexor group saw hot flashes increase; this did not happen with the acupuncture group. Most women in the latter group reported an improvement in energy, clarity of thought and sense of well-being and one-quarter experienced increased sex drive, all without the side effects (dizziness and anxiety) of Effexor.

Reiki is an ancient Tibetan healing energy system rediscovered by a Japanese monk in the 19th century. "Reiki" means universal life force energy similar to "chi" in Chinese healing or "prana" in yoga. It is believed to work on all levels — mental, physical, emotional and spiritual — in order to amplify people's innate abilities to heal themselves. In many studies, patients who received reiki treatments before chemotherapy reported a decrease in post-chemo reactions; others reported a dramatic reduction in pain levels, greater sense of calmness and peace when dealing with pain.

Relaxation training has been shown to be of benefit to women who had been treated for breast cancer and were suffering bothersome hot flashes. One hundred and fifty patients were recruited for a relaxation study. The first group was assigned to **relaxation training**; the second group verbally discussed traditional hot flash management suggestions with a nurse, but received no specific therapy.

Women in the relaxation group were given a session in deep breathing, muscle release and guided imagery. They took home audiotapes so they could repeat the session on their own. Over the next three months, women in both groups kept track of their hot flash symptoms in a diary.

After the first month, the researchers found that women in the relaxation group were reporting fewer and less severe hot flash episodes and also reported lower distress levels than the discussion-only group.

Why Good Sleep is So Important

Sleep is just as important to your overall health and longevity as good nutrition, sufficient exercise and the ability to manage your emotions and the stress of daily life — just ask anyone who has been sleep-deprived for more than a couple of nights. Did you realize that light, noise, electromagnetic fields, and movement in your bed not made by you all have the potential to disturb your sleep?

Insufficient, poor quality sleep can undermine all your other efforts to lead a healthy lifestyle and can contribute to some very serious conditions, including:

- Weakened immune system
- Faster tumour growth
- Increased risk of cancer, heart disease, diabetes, and obesity

There are many articles giving tips on getting good sleep habits. Pay special attention to melatonin production and elimination of electronic devices in the bedroom. So be sure to get those ZZZZZZZZZZZZZZZs! And review the message about melatonin in chapter 2.

Healing the Emotions

Find a place inside where there is joy and the joy will burn out the pain.

Joseph Campbell

Who can describe the fear and pain the diagnosis of any major illness can bring? For most women, breast cancer strikes at the very core of our roles as nurturers. Studies have shown that we can choose the thoughts that will change our emotions.

There are many studies supporting the belief that people with an upbeat and positive perspective tend to be healthier and enjoy longer lives. Despair and hopelessness raise the risk of heart attacks and cancer, just as joy and fulfillment keep us healthy and extend life. Recent widows are twice as likely to develop breast cancer. Distressed mental states get converted into bio-chemicals that create disease. And just as these mental states can create disease, they can also reverse the process and contribute to a return to good health.

Transcendental Meditation is a completely natural and comforting practice known to reduce stress and improve the emotional and mental well-being of practitioners. New studies suggest that **TM** offers the foundation of strength and inner peace so necessary to promote healing and recovery in breast cancer patients.

Music therapy also supports cancer patients to improve both emotional and physical well-being. Music therapy may accompany medical treatment to promote wellness, manage stress, alleviate pain and enhance memory. Music has been shown to help patients communicate and express feelings, and even promote physical rehabilitation. A physical response to music can also relax muscles and dilate veins, both of which can make procedures less uncomfortable.

A study from University of Montreal researchers stressed out participants (gave them math to do in front of an audience). During a break, half were given music to listen to and half sat in a silent room. Only the music listeners did not experience a spike in cortisol levels.

In studies of breast cancer patients, guided imagery has been shown to strengthen the immune system and enhance the ability to heal, relieve anxiety, and depression, as well as decrease side effects and complications of medical procedures. **Guided imagery,** sometimes known as **"visualization,"** is a technique in which a person imagines pictures, sounds, smells, and other sensations associated with reaching a goal. Imagining being in a certain environment or situation can activate the senses, producing a physical or psychological effect.

Almost anyone can use this technique. Guided imagery can be practiced at home with a book or audio recording or with a trained therapist. Patients also learn how to create their own images and/ or use previously created tapes.

- Set a goal
- Create a clear idea or picture
- Focus on it often
- Give it positive energy

Published on **Nov 16, 2013 o**nline:

Here is a very beautiful guided visualization exercise for cancer patients at any stage of disease or wellness to facilitate your own natural immune response. Helps activate your Tumor Infiltrating Leukocytes and Natural Killer Cells while protecting your healthy cells. You will visualize that tumor cells will be powerless against your own body's natural healing resources. This visualization is appropriate whether you are about to begin treatment or have completed treatment long ago. 40 minutes long, works even if you fall asleep! **Please feel free to share with any cancer patient or survivor who could benefit from a guided meditation.**

http://www.youtube.com/watch?v=Qm_SVBCY58w

Visualization was a big part of my healing agenda. After reading *Dreamhealer*, I used imagery every evening before falling asleep. I knew the location of the tumor and concentrated on shrinking it. In my mind it was like a pearl in the oyster of my breast. I reversed the process of accumulative layers on the pearl, rejecting the negative fighting mode. I rallied the T-cells to perform this mission which was a dissolving action. By imagining the layers melting and being carried away to be eliminated in the urine, the tumor became smaller.

Earlier in the evening I would listen to a self-healing hypnosis recording which put me into a very relaxed mood and summoned my innate healing energies, surrounding me with healing light and positive thoughts.

To this day, I use visualization whenever I feel any dis-ease taking hold, fully believing that I am shortening recovery time.

Breastcancer.org cites a Korean study (2005) in which 30 breast cancer patients were given **progressive muscle realization therapy** (PMRT) and taught to use **guided imagery** during their six months of **chemotherapy**. Another 30 were treated with chemo alone. The first group experienced less nausea and vomiting and members were less anxious, depressed and irritable than those receiving chemo alone. Six months after treatment ended, the PMRT and guided imagery group was still experiencing a better quality of life than the group that did not receive training.
17 June 2015 < http://www.breastcancer.org/treatment/comp_med/types/imagery

Journaling is creating a written account of events and emotions. Many healthcare clinics are suggesting journaling as a method to cope with serious illness.

Any major illness is an emotionally taxing experience. Journaling has been shown to increase a patient's coping mechanisms. Getting feelings on paper is a relief of stress, helps the patient to cope and plays a direct role in improving health. In addition, journaling can benefit psychologically through gaining insight and understanding of experiences. It's also a concrete measure of progress and a record of events and procedures.

Tips to get started:

- Find a quiet space and get in touch with what is bothering you
- Write continuously for a set amount of time
- Write about both events and feelings
- Provide as many details as possible
- Don't worry about spelling and grammar, just let it flow
- Don't stop until the allotted time is up

A **gratitude journal**, as recommended by Oprah Winfrey, can help one to stay in the moment and be focussed on the blessings in life. Positive entries and affirmations recorded daily in a handsome book can be kept for future reference and act as reminders. The negatives recorded separately on filing cards, once recognized, can then be consciously discarded and released.

Start each day by thinking of all the things you have to be thankful for; remember that your future depends largely on the thoughts you think *today*. So each moment of every day is an opportunity to turn your thinking around and feel more positive in the very next moment. Focus on the present moment and realize that each moment is good *right now*. You can practice gratitude by committing random acts of kindness, even it's only a smile to a stranger or an encouraging remark to an overworked cashier, a compliment to a harassed young mother.

Researchers have shown that when people engage in humour-associated mirthful **laughter**, their brain wave frequencies are similar to that which are seen when a person engages in meditation. Mirthful laughter has been shown to improve immune function and decrease stress levels.

Perhaps one of the most well-known forerunners of "the science of happiness" was Norman Cousins, who in 1964 was diagnosed with a life-threatening autoimmune disease. After being given a one in 500 chance of recovery, Cousins created his own **laughter therapy** program, which he claims was the key to his ultimate recovery.

Laughter Yoga is a unique form of exercise that was founded in 1995 by, a medical doctor from Mumbai, India. Dr. Madan Kataria, and his wife developed a program that combines laughter as a physical and playful body exercise with yoga in the form of deep yogic breathing (no poses).

Laughter yoga increases oxygen to the body and brain, enhances health, promotes joy and even World Peace. It is a great exercise for people of all ages and provides a sense of well-being. What started as one group of 5 people in a park in Mumbai in 1995, has now grown to become a worldwide phenomenon with more than 8000 clubs in over 79 countries.

See my good friend Kathryn Kimmins, Certified Laughter Yoga Instructor's website for more information: http://www. laughyourselfhealthy.ca/

But then again:

According to the Oprah doctors Oz and Roizen, when you shed emotional tears, in moments of intense feeling, they carry and wash away stress hormones. The urge to cry also signals that you've reached a level of stress that's bad for your health. Showing your vulnerability to friends can help also soothe the bad effects of stress. Tears are good for you, so go ahead and cry if you feel the need. Just as sweat removes salt, tears have a purpose, too.

Aromatherapy is the practice of using essential oils, usually from plants, to change a person's mood or to improve health. Essential oils are extracted from plants using different methods. The oils are usually very fragrant and highly concentrated.

- ➤ Take slow deep breaths through your nose to enhance the power of fragrance stress fighters.
- ➤ Lavender has long been recognized for its relaxation benefits. A study published in *Stress and Health* reveals that people who regularly breathe in peppermint essential oils are even less stressed (with lower cortisol levels) than those who use lavender.
- ➤ Lemon is an instant mood booster.

Aromatherapy is often used as a complementary therapy along with conventional cancer treatment to improve a person's quality of life. There is strong evidence that some types of essential oils may help:

- ▪ reduce stress
- ▪ promote a sense of calm or well-being
- ▪ lessen pain
- ▪ relieve nausea
- ▪ promote sleep

Read more: <http://www.cancer.ca/en/cancer-information/diagnosis-and-treatment/complementary-herapies/aromatherapy>

I was so impressed by the therapeutic benefits of essential oils that I became a distributer for doTerra, "certified pure therapeutic grade" essential oils.

Dr. Edward Bach developed **Flower Essence Therapy** in the 1930s. There are 38 flower essences made from non-poisonous plants, trees, and shrubs. Flower essence remedies are unique in that they work on a vibrational level to help release energy blocks between one's personality and their Higher Self. Flower essence remedies bring about the necessary changes in one's outlook that allows them to attain optimal health and wellness of mind, body, and spirit. They do not interact or interfere with medications or supplements and are complementary to all other healing modalities.

Healing with the Mind

No problem can be solved from the same level of consciousness that created it.

Albert Einstein

How mysterious is the world of the internet! On this invisible web, everything is linked and available for our research and expanding knowledge, for reaching out and seeing others at a distance, for connecting to lives and events from long ago. Just as wondrous and mysterious are the latest theories of quantum physics, indicating everything is related to an invisible force and energy. You and I are pure energy-light in a beautiful and intelligent form.

Nothing is solid and all our thoughts are linked to this invisible energy. It is our thoughts that determine the form that energy manifests. Your thoughts literally shift the universe to create your physical life. The constantly changing energy beneath the surface of your physical body is controlled with your powerful mind.

One thing I learned long ago, and I consider to be one of the most important lessons of my life, is that I can choose which thoughts to entertain. My mind cannot hold two thoughts at one time and when faced with a negative worry or a positive affirmation, I have the choice to eliminate the self-destructive thought and to be encouraged by the positive one. This has helped me through many difficult situations. Try it; control your own thoughts! Do not let your thoughts control you.

"A fundamental conclusion of the new physics also acknowledges that the observer creates the reality. As observers, we are personally involved with the creation of our own reality. Physicists are being forced to admit that the universe is a 'mental' construction."
R. C. Henry, "The Mental Universe"; Nature 436:29, 2005, Professor of Physics and Astronomy at Johns Hopkins University:

In the September 12, 2004, *Dallas Morning News*, scientists from the University of Texas Southwestern Medical Center at Dallas reported that not only do cells have memory, but whether their memories are positive or negative can mean the difference between health and disease, even life and death.

And:
"All matter is energy."
Albert Einstein

"All living organisms emit an energy field."
Semyon Kirlian, USSR

"The energy field starts it all."
Prof. Harold Burr, PhD, Yale University

"Body chemistry is covered by quantum cellular fields."
Prof. Murray Gell-Mann, Nobel Prize Laureate (1969)

"Diseases are to be diagnosed and prevented via energy field assessment."
George Crile, Sr. M.D. Founder of the Cleveland Clinic

"Treating humans without the concept of energy is treating dead matter."
Albert Szent-Gyorgyi, MD, Nobel Laureate (1937), Hungary

and
..."The root of all health and illness is always an energy issue in the body."
Dr. Alex Loyd; http://www.thehealingcodeinfo.com/

The Healing Code focuses on the spiritual issues of the heart, believing "that the energy frequency of pure love will heal anything -- and that may be the only power that will."

"In 2001 Dr. Alex Loyd discovered how to activate a physical function built into the body so that the neuro-immune system takes over its job of healing whatever is wrong in the body. His findings were validated scientifically and by the thousands of people from all over the world who have used *The Healing Codes*® system to heal virtually any physical, emotional, or relational issue, as well as realize breakthroughs in success."

You can also use *The Healing Code* to heal other people. The book gives instructions for how to do *The Healing Code* on behalf of another person. Just as you would pray for another person, so you can do *The Healing Code* for someone with cancer, diabetes, arthritis, MS, or a difficult relationship issue. Distance is not an issue, any more than it is a problem to pray for someone who is not physically present with you.

In *Chasing the Cure*, William Bengston recounts his experiments with energy healing. In 10 separate trials where clinical animals were injected with a lethal strain of mammary cancer, 90% were cured with hands-on healing. The studies were conducted in four different labs in the US and results were published in peer-reviewed journals.

Said Sylvia Fraser, Hamilton–born co-author of *Chasing the Cure*: "Bill simply blew me away with his research and his proof."

<http://www.bengstonresearch.com/>

Spiritual Healing

Your pain is the breaking of the shell that encloses your understanding.
Kahlil Gibran

Prayer

Prayer is letting go of the belief you are in charge of your life and giving it over to something more inclusive than your own point of view; it requires a leap of faith.

And the prayer of faith will save the one who is sick, and the Lord will raise him up. And if he has committed sins, he will be forgiven.

Therefore, confess your sins to one another and pray for one another, that you may be healed. The prayer of a righteous person has great power as it is working. James 5:15-16

Research focusing on the power of prayer in healing has nearly doubled in the past 10 years.

Even the NIH (National Institutes of Health) is now funding one prayer study through its Frontier Medicine Initiative.

Dr. Mehmet Oz has spoken on his television show about the power of prayer. Dr. Oz said he has seen a number of miracles as a doctor and, on his program, he invited an expert in this area. Dr. Harold Koenig, a physician who believes in the power of prayer, is a professor of psychiatry at Duke University. He's done a lot of research to connect medicine and spirituality to find out the link between prayer and health.

Dr. Koenig said that people, who are spiritual but not religious, derive benefit from meditation. But when people pray within the context of talking to God, it seems to make a difference.

Prayer has even helped Dr. Koenig manage years of chronic pain in his own life. He says that people who are religious lead healthier lives and can add 7 to 10 years to their lifespan.

Dr. Wayne Dyer, renowned spiritual writer and lecturer, credits John of God, spiritual healer in Brazil, with his distance healing of leukemia. His death in 2015 was attributed to heart attack, not his leukemia which was still in remission.

Praying takes the mind off worrying

Elizabeth Lesser *New York Times* best-selling author of *The Seeker's Guide* and *Broken Open*:

"My favorite advice about prayer from Sister Alice is this: 'If you are going to pray, then don't worry. And if you are going to worry, then don't bother praying. You can't be doing both.' When I stop and listen closely to what's going on inside my head, I often hear the buzz of worry, like the drone of bees in a wall. That's when I remember Sister Alice's words of wisdom. What would I rather be doing, I ask myself, worrying or praying? I usually choose praying. It's a lot more fun than worrying."

Elizabeth Kubler-Ross is best known as the medical doctor who co-founded the hospice movement around the world. She was also the author of the ground-breaking book *On Death and Dying*, which first discussed The Five Stages of Grief. Her faith in prayer is legendary.

"You will not grow if you sit in a beautiful flower garden, but you will grow if you are sick, if you are in pain, if you experience losses, and if you do not put your head in the sand, but take the pain as a gift to you with a very, very specific purpose."

The only thing we can really ask for when we pray is the ability to trust in that greater purpose. We pray to have our hearts opened and our purpose revealed.

Read more: www.oprah.com/spirit/ what-Prayer-Really-Means-Elizabeth-Lesser/2>

Labyrinths are ancient, sacred patterns that combine the imagery of the circle and the spiral into a meandering but purposeful path. Labyrinths have long been used as meditation and prayer tools. Many people walk the labyrinth as an effective and pleasurable way to practice mindfulness, bringing awareness into the present moment and connecting one to nature. It is becoming very common for hospitals to install **labyrinths** within their walls or on their grounds for patient and staff use.

How to Live in the Moment
http://www.wikihow.com/Live-in-the-Moment

- Living in the moment is all about living like there's no tomorrow. To do this, you must realize beauty in every moment and in everyday activities. It's a conscious act that requires participation, not just observation. This is your life, now live!
- Be optimistic.
- To live in the moment, to "dance like nobody's watching," you have to forget about performing for others and simply accept the moment for what it is.
- Take notice of the world around you. No matter what you're doing, notice the moments that surround you: a beautiful vista, a view of the sunrise, the colours of changing leaves. Really look at a flower. Realizing that whether these things are great or small, you are part of that singular moment when all these things come together.
- Focus on whatever you're doing. Even if you're just walking, or folding clothes, or shuffling cards—how does it feel? There's probably some kind of commentary spinning through your mind, and it probably has to do with something other than what you're doing. Let those thoughts go and focus on what is (not what was, or what could be). In Buddhism, this is referred to as mindfulness.
- Just breathe. When the moment begins to escape you, as it will certainly try to do, breathe. Take a very deep breath,

through your nose, as deep as you can. Breathe out slowly through your mouth, letting the air escape on its own.

- Pay attention to your other senses—touch, sight, smell, sound, and taste. Have you ever been so engrossed in something that it seemed like the rest of the world just disappeared? Living in the moment is about creating that state of mind at any time. Slow down, and try to savor the present.

- Listen to the world. The birds, the ticking of a clock (when you are lucky to encounter one that ticks), the planes overhead, the footsteps of passers-by. The moment is all around you.

- Smile when you wake up. You can set the tone of appreciation and awareness for the next 24 hours. There's scientific proof that the expressions that you make with your face can actually influence how you feel.

- Commit random, spontaneous acts of kindness. Keep alert in every moment of your day for some way in which you can make the world a better place. Even the smallest thing, such as complimenting someone, can bring joy to you as well as the other person.

- Be thankful for what is. When you find yourself wishing for something you don't have, or wishing your life would be different, start your quest for your wish by being thankful for what is already in your life. This will bring you back to the present moment.

- Make a list of what you are thankful for right now, even if all you can think of is that you are alive and can breathe. You don't want to miss the gifts right in front of you, because you are always looking beyond what is in the present moment to what once was or what might be. If you are thankful for what is, you'll be happy to be in the moment – instead of dreaming about being happy someplace else.

"Article provided by wikiHow, a wiki building the world's largest, highest quality how-to manual. Content on wikiHow can be shared under a Creative Commons License."

A Zen tale about living in the moment:

There was once a man who was being chased by a ferocious tiger across a field. At the edge of the field there was a cliff. In order to escape the jaws of the tiger, the man caught hold of a vine and swung himself over the edge of the cliff. That's when he noticed a wild strawberry growing on the cliff wall. Clutching the vine with one hand, he plucked the succulent berry and popped it into his mouth exclaiming: "how delicious."

New study findings suggest **Transcendental Meditation** reduces stress and improves the emotional and mental well-being of breast cancer patients.

Pay attention to your dreams

All through the ages, dreams have been regarded as the language of the soul. Our subconscious mind sends us messages (if we can remember and interpret them!). With conscious effort you can remember more of your dreams and recall them in greater detail.

- Put a pad and pen or pencil within easy reach of your bed.
- Calm your mind and body before bedtime.
- Make a conscious decision to remember your dreams.
- Repeat three times: "I will remember my dreams".
- Concentrate on recalling your dream as soon as you wake up.

- Record your dream in your dream journal immediately upon awakening, before doing anything else.
- Be careful about interpreting dreams; for example, a dream about death does not mean that someone will die, or that something bad will happen.

March 3

> *Operation was Feb. 22. Breast dream was Feb. 12, 2005. I dreamed I had a third breast growing under my right arm. I should have paid attention – at that point it was stage one, but because it was a "breast" not cancer in my dream, I know all will be well. It is amazing to me how I do not fear or worry. I simply know all will be well. This is the true gift of faith. It is simply a gift that I am grateful for. I have received so much love and attention—calls prayers and flowers. Andrea stayed 2 nights – away from her wonderful baby Matty. Tom called 2x and sent flowers. We laughed and laughed today – so therapeutic.*

Healers Worth Noting and Worth Knowing About

Rene Caisse, Canada's Cancer Nurse 1887 - 1978

In 1922 when Rene Caisse was a nurse in Haileybury, Ontario, she met an elderly woman whose breast cancer had earlier been sent into remission by an Ojibwa medicine man whose only remedy was a concoction of four herbs: burdock root, sheep sorrel, slippery elm bark, and turkey rhubarb root. Caisse experimented on laboratory mice by treating tumors with her "Essiac," the herbal remedy which is an anagram of her surname.

Her first test case was her mother's sister. After consultation with her aunt's doctor and under his watchful supervision, Rene treated her aunt, who was dying of stomach cancer. Her aunt obtained full remission and lived another 21 years. Her aunt's doctor asked Rene to treat still other cancer patients. Soon other physicians began sending their cancer patients to her. Eight of these doctors petitioned the Department of Health and Welfare in Ottawa to give nurse Caisse "an opportunity to prove her work in a big way." This petition was dated at Toronto on October 27, 1926.

Dr. Frederick Banting, the co-discoverer of insulin, used his influence to petition the University of Toronto to give Rene access to laboratory facilities for her research. However, since the formula for Essiac would become exclusively the University's, Nurse Caisse balked. She did not want her secret formula taken out of the public good and locked away. Hauled before the courts for practicing without a license, she produced, for all her patients, scripts duly authorized by their attending physicians.

On December 23, 1936, a group of doctors petitioned Queen's Park: "... we, the undersigned do strongly urge that the ... Minister of Health take immediate action, to make this treatment [Essiac] available for cancer sufferers, and keep it a Canadian discovery."

In 1938, a private member's bill was proposed as "an Act to authorize Rene Caisse to practice medicine in the Province of Ontario in the treatment of Cancer...." The Bill was signed by 55 thousand persons in favour of its passage, including 387 patients. Many of the signatories were doctors.

Before a vote was taken, the government set up a Royal Cancer Commission. Over 2000 documented cases of cancer cures came forward, but only 49 were reviewed. The final verdict:

"not enough evidence was found to substantiate the claims of Essiac." Because Essiac was not government-approved as a drug-related treatment for cancer, nurse Caisse closed her clinic in 1942 fearing slander, lawsuits and – ultimately – jail. Rene Caisse always refused monetary payment for her services stating: "The love and respect of my fellow man means more than riches." However, mainstream medicine continued to portray her as a misguided simpleton touting a "witch doctor's brew." She never did turn her herbal formula over to any authorities. No one, through scientific experiment, ever proved that her herbal tea does not work. Her legacy lies in the fact that today thousands of people are still using the Essiac formula with some success.

In 1959, the story of Essiac and Nurse Rene Caisse, then in her 70s, attracted the attention of Charles Brusch, M.D., John F. Kennedy's personal physician and the first doctor in the U.S. to administer polio vaccine as well as the doctor after whom the world-famous Brusch Medical Centre in Boston is named. Caisse entered into an agreement with Brusch and the Medical Centre to research Essiac. After Rene died in 1978, Dr. Brusch still administered Essiac to patients, claiming Essiac even cured his own colon cancer in 1984.

Reprinted with permission *from Visionaries: Canadian Triumphs*, Heirloom Publishing, Mississauga Ontario, 1998

DREAMHEALER

Dr. Adam McLeod is a Naturopathic Doctor, molecular biologist, internationally renowned First Nations energy healer and best-selling author. As a teenager, Adam's healing of celebrity Ronnie Hawkins of pancreatic cancer led to world-wide recognition and acclaim.

Over the last 10 years Adam has been credited with hundreds of healings from those who have read his books and attended his workshops. At these workshops he bridges his innate healing abilities with naturopathic knowledge to teach others how to access their own healing abilities to become self-empowered.

For updated schedule of workshops see:

http://dreamhealer.com/workshop/

May 9, 2011

> *Attended Adam's workshop in Toronto with Alexandrea. During both healings (although ostensibly I was there to heal 'Andrea's diabetes) we were instructed to heal ourselves. I felt the urge to concentrate on my pineal gland and directed energy there.*

> ***Definition:*** *The pineal gland is part of the endocrine system. A small cone-shaped organ located in the cerebrum, the pineal gland produces the hormone melatonin, which regulates the sleep/wake cycle. Additionally, the pineal gland helps regulate blood pressure, body temperature, motor function, growth and sexual development.*

> *Today, Monday my FBS (fasting blood sugar) is 3.8 and BP (blood pressure) is 102/ 70 – neither has EVER been that low that low! So I will eliminate meds for today and see what happens. Bought the DVD to share as needed.*

> *My own notes from that workshop:*

> - *Treat the cause not the symptoms*
> - *Heal the whole person*

- *Reduce stress to heal: high levels of stress hormone compromise the immune system*
- *Be positive, relaxed and focussed on healing*
- *Environment directly affects expression of DNA, RNA and proteins*
- *Proteins affect virtually every aspect of metabolism; smallest change in environment affects proteins in subtle interaction*
- *Whatever you believe, use it to advantage: use intention to guide emotions.*
- *Emotions can be used to positively influence healing process e.g. positive memory creates duplicate feelings of the event.*
- *Be patient; healing is a process; it takes time*
- *Every single cell stores memory and emotion*
- *Practice positive visualizations and forgiveness*
- *Practice meditation daily; become aware of breath*
- *Maintain a journal*
- *Tap into circadian rhythm; do visualizations before falling asleep*
- *Set goals; focus intention and align conscious intention with subconscious thought*
- *basic steps:*
  - *Understand the problem*
  - *Understand body's mechanism for healing itself*
  - *Understand what perfect health looks like*
  - *Know your intentions are doing this to your body*
  - *Integrate your unique history and emotions to customize your visualizations: memories, events, hobbies, passions: use what resonates strongly with you – nobody knows YOU better than YOU*

Chapter 4

Surround, Pamper and Celebrate Yourself

When someone you love faces a personal challenge you probably wish you could help in some way. Remember how it helps to alleviate your concern to know you are doing something for a friend. So, to honour them also, allow others the privilege of helping you.

Family and friends not only serve as emotional support, they also help you decide which kind of surgery and treatment to have.

If you feel the need, be sure to call Cancer Societies and join support groups and perhaps volunteer with them when it is all behind you. You will be an expert survivor and may wish to share your experience and offer support to someone who is on the threshold of the maze that so bewilders and bewitches you now.

But in the long run, YOU are in charge when it comes to your health care – it's YOUR body!

- Trust and listen to your body; your body knows what is best for you

- Tune into your intuition
- Express your emotions
- Accept love and accept help
- Embrace illness for the lessons it teaches you
- Be open to messages from others (especially angels)

Put Yourself First

According to Dr. Cristiane Northrup, women who tend to be most at risk for breast cancer are those who have difficulty nurturing themselves and receiving pleasure. Nurturing self-love and self-acceptance is an important part of creating optimal health, especially for women.

So pay attention to your emotions and needs. Rest when you need to and pre-occupy or shift your thoughts with distracting, interesting activities. If possible, develop a new creative activity or rekindle one from the past.

Take time to look at the circumstances and events that are changing as a result of diagnosis. Social isolation can change the expression of genes important in the growth of mammary gland tumors.

Depending on your circumstances, you may decide to take time off from work or not. At this time, work is not your priority – you are! If your employer is not understanding and supportive, it may be time to find a new one — after you are healed. Do you really want to work for someone so inconsiderate?

When the ordeal is over you will realize that "this happened for a reason" which may or may not reveal itself to you for some time. But there IS a reason.

Investigate this further:

- Have I been giving and giving and giving care to others without caring for me?
- Am I unhappy in some area of life that I do not address?
- Is there a relationship that will become more whole as a result of this journey? Or diminish?
- Is this a wake-up call to take care of ME?
- Is this an opportunity to learn compassion for others less fortunate?
- Have I taken for granted some of the more important aspects of life?

Stress can adversely impact cancer. One study found stressful marriages are bad for breast cancer recovery. The implication is that perceived or actual stress from outside can affect which genes get turned on or off.

Cancer Prevention Research, Oct. 2009

When disclosing your situation to family and friends and colleagues, look into the eyes of the person to determine how you will deliver the message. Some will want details, some will want updates verbally by phone, others text or email updates. Some will not be comfortable with the conversation and should be allowed to lead the way in discussions for details.

So first of all, be your own best friend. Treat yourself as you would care for your daughter if she were facing surgery. After years of no self-pampering, I found that manicures and pedicures, Reiki treatments and massages were soothing time-fillers. And what a pleasure to see what grooming self-improvement can do for attitude!

Cancer survivor Debbie Watters wrote *Where's Mom's Hair?* a book to address the fears children face when a parent is diagnosed with cancer. Touching and humorous black and white photographs follow Mom (Debbie) as she and her family go through each step of fighting cancer. And, for your husband's insight and understanding there is *Breast Cancer Husband* by Marc Silver.

◇◇

In prosperity our friends know us; in adversity we know our friends.
John Churton Collins

In some cases you may find that friends do not live up to the title and you may consider dropping those relationships. Many times, casual acquaintances will reveal new depths to be cultivated further.

To make it easier for you and your family and friends, prepare a "helping hands" list of things that would help you or your family such as:

- Preparing a meal
- Cutting the grass
- Driving the kids to activities
- Shopping for groceries
- Joining you on an appointment
- Taking you out for a coffee visit

When someone asks how can I help? Use the list!
Keep all information in one place. Make your wishes known.

Suggestions for concerned friends:

- Don't wait to be asked to do something. See what needs to be done; help will be appreciated
- Instead of flowers send a home-cooked meal, pizza or fruit basket
- Offer to pick up groceries
- Offer rides to and from appointments
- Watch for opportunities to talk about feelings and experiences. Don't push if your friend does not wish to share
- Give:
    - Easy-to-care for plants which represent life
    - Funny movies because "laughter is the best medicine"
    - Gift certificates for yoga and laughter yoga
    - Spa gift certificates
    - Inspirational books
    - Favourite music CDs

Feb. 7
I am still optimistic and sure this is a transitional experience. Just want to get it over with!
I am overjoyed with response of friends. It feels so good. I am being loving and gentle with myself. Not pushing or rushing, just pampering. Early to bed, vitamins and reading.
Grateful for so many things. Soon to learn Reiki finally.
Amazed I do not worry about money. I just know it will come.

June 6

It was my birthday and the last day of my radiation treatments.

I sat alone among strangers, all with companions engaging them in conversations, for the last in a series of 17 treatments over a three-and-a-half week period.

I looked around and wondered why my stubbornly persistent independence streak had prevented me from asking anyone to accompany me over the course of therapy. Perhaps because it was my birthday, I felt a little sorry for myself.

Then, looking up from my self-absorbing thoughts, almost through a haze, I saw an angel approaching me.

Strolling down the corridor, red rose in hand, was Sylvia, my childhood friend – indeed a friend from infancy as our parents were close friends at the time of our three-weeks-apart births!

Sylvia's beautiful, radiant smile lit up the somber waiting space and all eyes turned her way as she hugged and kissed me "Happy Birthday". We reconnected for coffee after the treatment session and I was presented with a loving card and gift of a cherished pearl bracelet and a crystal bracelet with a pink ribbon charm.

This will always remain with me as one of the best birthdays of my life. I had finished the race and was acknowledged and indulged with beauty and grace in the beautiful form of friendship and love.

And THAT was most healing of all.

I know my journey was alleviated by the loving presence and support of dear, cherished family and friends. I bless them every day and count them as my most precious gifts.

Pampering and treating yourself may not be easy (but then again, maybe it will). In any case, it is an essential necessity to speed your recovery. It is an expression of self-love and most of us must learn to love ourselves better. Are you not aware that this is fundamental to truly loving someone else!

Be gentle with yourself. Give YOU permission to be indulgent – in beauty treatments, relaxation, time off, massages, mani's and pedi's, facials, any small indulgencies. Treat YOU as you would treat a favourite sister who is going through a rough time. The positive effect that little pamperings will have on your psyche will help the medicine go down more easily. You'll receive gifts of lotions, bath salts, spa gift certificates and so on. Use them and enjoy with gusto.

It is important to keep self-confidence and esteem high. For many women, hair loss is the most devastating effect of cancer treatment. The good news is this hair loss is temporary. Cancer treatment can also affect your skin, nails and oral health. Investing in a wig and beautiful headscarves goes a long way in boosting self-esteem.

Monica bought me the vitamin supplement Biotin and what a difference that made to my thinning hair and brittle nails! I still use it every day for added nutrients.

You can take charge of how you look and feel during your cancer journey.

Look Good Feel Better is an organization offering beauty and wellness tips specifically for women with cancer. On their website, you can learn how to choose a wig or tie a headscarf and recreate the look of lost eyebrows: easy techniques that will help you reclaim your sense of self so you can face cancer with confidence. There are many tips and information to help you look and feel more like yourself until your hair grows back.
http://lgfb.ca

After mastectomy, a wide variety of undergarments can renew femininity. Professional fitters can assist with proper, flattering styles of to accommodate lifestyle needs. and fit using full or partial breast forms.

Rethink Breast Cancer offers age-appropriate support in many areas for young women affected by breast cancer and uses donations to fund innovated education, research and support programs.

Their mission: to continuously pioneer cutting-edge breast cancer education, support and research that speaks fearlessly to the unique needs of young (or youngish) women http://rethinkbreastcancer.com/

In addition to your oncologist, a coach can help you understand and manage your disease. Patients are hiring cancer coaches to give a crash course, go to appointments with them, provide information about treatments and design diet and exercise programs.

PRO-HEALTH Coaching provides coaches to teach about the disease, guide patients through the complicated health care system, provide emotional support and fill in gaps in traditional treatment such as diet and exercise.

Wellwood, associated with the Juravinski Cancer Clinic in Hamilton, Ontario, offers 25 programs including peer support to "share the wisdom gathered from the experience of those who live and work with cancer to ease the journey for all".
www.wellwood.ca

Canadian Cancer Society also matches patients over the phone with a trained volunteer who has been through a similar experience.
1-(888) 939-3333

The volunteer service **Nanny Angel Network** provides volunteers up to five hours per week to give a break to moms undergoing breast cancer treatment.

The **Weekend to End Women's Cancer Walk** benefits the Princess Margaret Cancer Centre in Toronto and Montreal's Jewish General Hospital. This is an opportunity to meet and kibitz with many like-minded people.
http://www.endcancer.ca/

I was touched when a friend, Catherine, did the 60 km cancer walk over two days to raise funds for cancer research.

Since my own experience, I have resolved and generally adhere to using my "best" china, crystal, silverware and linens, even though I live and dine alone most of the time. Who am I saving it for? My younger generations do not find joy in the same accoutrements I once prized so highly.

Every day was a lesson in living in the moment. Pre-surgery, I regarded my pamperings as preparation; post-surgery, they were necessary and welcomed respites. I gave myself permission to relax, to read for pleasure, and to have cherished conversational visits with long-neglected friends. I created a **vision board** – a collage of images, pictures and affirmations of dreams and things that inspire happiness – and saw many of my long-held wishes come true.

Create a Vision Board

Decide the main theme of your board based on something specific you wish to accomplish or obtain (like continued good health and fitness), or it may be a general mood or collection of everything that makes you happy.

1. Find pictures from magazines that correspond with your subject.
2. Type or write some affirmations or quotations corresponding with your theme.
3. Arrange the pictures and affirmations in a pleasing collage on poster or cork board.
4. Secure your arrangement with glue or pins.
5. Hang your vision board in a place where you will see every day.
6. View your board at least once a day and focus on the objects, sayings and theme.

Vision boards really do bring dreams to reality. Imagine my surprise when, on a last minute trip to Spain, I found myself, on a day trip completely unplanned for, overlooking the exact scene, cut from a travel magazine, that I had been looking at on my vision board for over a year!

My dear friend, Leytha, attracted her darling husband after creating her dream board.

What long-held wishes and desires will your dream board manifest for you?

July 8, 2007

> *I am mentally prepared to leave all health problems behind me. Will job search in earnest; write my book. Lots of family news: a wedding (Jamie and Cheryl) and new baby (Alexandrea and Ilo) to look forward to. Planning a trip to Greece via Greg's air miles.*
>
> *Today, (six months after diagnosis) I was sure I had my energy back: cooking, baking (banana bread) shopping, making dinner, cleaning-up etc.*
> *There is so much to be grateful for!*

So now, THAT part of my journey was complete; phase 2 is the rest of my life! With my awareness on high-alert, there are definite, proven life-style adaptations for me to follow that can ensure the next third will be healthy and cancer-free.

Chapter 5

Welcome a New Self

Like most women, I had always believed that I would escape cancer of any kind let alone breast cancer. After all, according to several friends, I did everything "right". I ate a low fat (but not anymore, having happily added healthy fats), nutritionally-conscious diet, slept well, exercised (albeit very moderately) and had never smoked. My lifestyle bordered on boring! I had a lot to learn about this mysterious interloper that took over my life and altered it forever!

Cancer has been around as long as mankind, but in the second half of the 20th century the number of cases seems to have exploded. Contributing to the ever-increasing number of cancer diagnoses are the extreme amounts of toxins and pollutants that we are exposed to, high stress lifestyles that tax the immune system, poor quality junk food, everyday food that is full of pesticides, irradiated and now genetically modified (GMO), pathogens, electromagnetic stress, artificial lighting, and everything electronic that our modern lifestyle dictates we must own. The list goes on and on!

All these factors weaken the immune system and alter the internal environment in the body to create a situation that promotes the growth of cancer. Cancer tumors begin when cancerous cells are being created at a rate greater than an overworked, depleted immune system can destroy.

It is normal to fear a recurrence of your breast cancer. According to National Cancer Institute nearly 7 out of 10 survivors worry about cancer returning. Your personal risk of recurrence will depend of a variety of factors, including your type of breast cancer, your treatment protocol and your genetics.

Cancer is not a mysterious disease that suddenly attacks you out of the blue, something that you can't do anything about. It has definite causes that can be corrected. You can change your internal environment to one that creates supportive health while at the same time attacks cancerous cells and tumors.

Thousands of studies show that **simple lifestyle strategies** can be tremendously protective against cancer. These strategies include boosting the immune system, with **food, supplements, herbs, exercise** and **avoiding toxic exposure**. I have summarized many of the studies that can help you decide which lifestyle changes are right for you. You probably will not adopt all of them; the important thing is to make small, frequent adaptations which will add up to a long lifetime of good health, not only preventing cancer recurrence but preventing other diseases as well and adding to enjoyment of quality of life in general.

Exercise

You cannot rely on healthy eating alone to protect you from certain cancers. **Exercise** is a must! (Yes, my dear, it is!) A series of studies have been published that link physical exercise to reduced breast cancer risk and increased survival. The March 2009 issue of the *Journal of Sports Sciences* reports that moderate or vigorous exercise reduced breast cancer risk by 44 per cent. An earlier study published in 2007 in the journal *Cancer Detection and Prevention* likewise showed that breast cancer risk was reduced by 40 per cent among women with moderate physical activity and 57 per cent with vigorous activity.

Breast cancer is the most common cancer in women. A woman's lifetime chance of getting breast cancer is about one in eight. Obese women are up to 60 percent more likely to develop any cancer than normal-weight women. Many breast cancers are fueled by estrogen, a hormone produced and stored in fat tissue. So experts suspect that the more overweight a woman is, the more estrogen she's likely to produce, which could eventually trigger breast cancer. Even in slim women, exercise can help reduce the cancer risk by converting more of the body's fat into muscle.

Researchers at a breast cancer conference (7th European Breast Cancer Conference, March 2010, Barcelona, Spain) reported that up to a third of breast cancer cases in western countries could be avoided if women ate less and exercised more and that the focus should shift to changing behaviors like diet and physical activity.

Physical exercise contributes a simple, non-invasive non-chemical, inexpensive means of cancer prevention. In most cases microscopic changes occur 10-15 years before breast cancer is discovered. But over time, exercise can delay those life-threatening changes. See facingcancer.ca for strength-building exercises.

Here's some good news that I was happy to read:
An article by Dr. Martin Gibala of Hamilton, Ontario's McMaster University concludes: "Just six minutes of intense exercise a week

does as much to improve a person's fitness as a regime of six hours." That intense workout was furious cycling.

Better to walk every day for half an hour, swim, do heavy gardening or housework, but exercise; that is the key. A cancer research centre showed that women who walked briskly for 2 hours each week reduced their risk by 18 per cent.

Nordic walking which employs wrist –height poles with straps for upper body workout has been recommended as the best exercise for breast cancer survivors.

Diet

Like exercise, **good nutrition** is a foundation of cancer prevention. An anti-cancer diet focusses on fiber-rich, unprocessed foods with a decreased intake of alcohol and processed meats. Breast cancer survival is improved when individuals consume high amounts of fiber: 21 to 38 grams are recommended.

High fiber foods include bran, broccoli, cabbage, berries, leafy greens, celery, squash, beans, lentils, mushrooms, and oranges. Individuals who increase their intake of fiber should also increase their intake of water.

Diabetes and obesity increase the risk of breast cancer as reported in a study presented by San Antonio Breast Cancer Symposium, December 11, 2011.

However, **Metformin,** the most common first-line drug in the treatment of type 2 diabetes, has been shown in studies to reduce breast cancer risk, improve survival rates and increase the effectiveness of chemotherapy.

Based on extensive laboratory research, **Metformin** is being tested in clinical trials not only as a treatment for cancer, but as a way to prevent it in people at increased risk, including cancer survivors who have a higher risk of a second primary cancer.

A higher consumption of refined carbohydrates (starches and sugars) results in a 50 per cent increased risk of recurrence. A study of 5450 post-menopausal women followed over 8 years measured blood sugar levels and insulin at 1, 3 and 6 years. Those with high insulin levels had double the risk of developing cancer. Those in the top third for insulin levels had triple the risk compared to those with lowest third.

Weight gain with every decade of life from age 18 roughly doubles the risk of cancer. However, even among lean women, having raised insulin levels significantly increases cancer risk. Insulin levels go up in response to a high glycemic load (GL) diet. The solution is to consume a low GL diet.

Acidic levels: There is plenty of research showing cancer thrives in an acidic environment and does not survive in a normal, more alkaline environment. Taking action to ensure your body is more alkaline is an important step in your battle against cancer. As mentioned elsewhere, meats, grains, sugar and soft drinks are acidic and should be used moderately.

I use a Santevia alkaline stick in my non-plastic water bottle to alkalinize my water. Drinking fresh lemon juice in warm water first thing in the morning is a good practice to alkalinize and detoxify your body.

Dr. Joseph Mercola named an "Ultimate Wellness Game Changer" by *Huffington Post* believes the vast majority of all cancers could be prevented by strictly applying the healthy lifestyle recommendations summarized below.

- **Avoid sugar**, especially fructose, and processed foods. All forms of sugar are detrimental to health in general and promote cancer. Refined fructose, however, is clearly one of the most harmful and should be avoided as much as possible. This automatically means avoiding processed foods, as most are loaded with fructose (typically in the form of high fructose corn syrup, HFCS).
- **Optimize your vitamin D levels**. Vitamin D influences virtually every cell in your body and is one of nature's most potent cancer fighters. Vitamin D is actually able to enter cancer cells and trigger apoptosis (cell death).
- **Limit your protein**. Newer research has emphasized the importance of the motor pathways. When these are active, cancer growth is accelerated. One way to quiet this pathway is by limiting your protein to one gram of protein per kilogram of lean body mass. For most people this ranges between 40 and 70 grams of protein a day, which is typically about 2/3 to half of what they are currently eating.
- **Avoid unfermented soy products**. Unfermented soy is high in plant estrogens, or phytoestrogens, also known as isoflavones.
- **Improve your insulin and leptin receptor sensitivity.** The best way to do this is by avoiding sugar and grains and restricting carbs to mostly fiber vegetables.
- **Exercise regularly.** One of the primary reasons exercise works to lower your cancer risk is because it drives your insulin levels down, and controlling your insulin levels is one

of the most powerful ways to reduce your cancer risks. It has also been suggested that apoptosis (programmed cell death) is triggered by exercise, causing cancer cells to die.

- **Maintain a healthy body weight**. It's important to lose excess body fat because fat produces estrogen.
- **Drink a pint to a quart of organic green vegetable juice daily.**
- **Get plenty of high-quality, animal-based omega-3 fats, such as fish and krill oil. Omega-3 deficiency** is a common underlying factor for cancer. Vegetarian choices include nuts and seeds.
- **Avoid drinking alcohol**, or at least limit your alcoholic drinks to one per day.
- **Avoid electromagnetic fields as much as possible.**
- **Avoid synthetic hormone replacement therapy (HRT), especially if you have risk factors for breast cancer.**
- **Avoid BPA, phthalates, and other xenoestrogens.**
- **Make sure you're not iodine deficient**, as there's compelling evidence linking iodine deficiency with certain forms of cancer. Iodine has potent anticancer properties and has been shown to cause cell death in breast and thyroid cancer cells.
- **Avoid charring your meats**.

The entire article, **Cancer Prevention Begins with Your Lifestyle Choices** can be found at **http://fitness.mercola.com/sites/fitness/archive/2012/11/30/exercise-protects-immune-system.aspx**

Antioxidants are man-made or natural substances that may prevent or delay some types of cell damage. ORACValues.com is a comprehensive database of foods and their antioxidant levels.

Reducing your sugar and fructose intake will decrease your antioxidant stress. So limit sugars and processed foods. You can also wisely select targeted nutrients to supplement your food choices.

Some very good immune-boosting foods are listed later in this chapter. To get the full list see http://www.oracvalues.com/

Preventing and Fighting Cancer

Plant-based foods are cancer-fighting powerhouses. The best diet for preventing or fighting cancer is a predominantly plant-based diet eating mostly foods that come from plants: vegetables, fruits, seeds, nuts, grains, and beans. Plants have less fat, more fiber, and more cancer-fighting nutrients. These three elements work together to support your immune system and help your body fight off cancer.

The less processed that foods are — that is, the less they've been cooked, peeled, mixed with other ingredients, stripped of their nutrients, or otherwise altered from the way they came out of the ground — the better. Also, consume locally-grown and organic foods where possible. Local and pesticide–free produce is better for you AND for the planet.

Have you noticed food no longer tastes like it used to? If you are a boomer-baby or older, you may recall how delicious garden tomatoes smelled and tasted before big-farm production with growth-enhancing chemicals and pesticides turned them into perfect-looking but tasteless blobs. How about the smell and flavor of farmer market fruits and vegetables before mass transportation from exotic countries? We are fortunate to have available so many "fresh" veggies and fruits all winter long, but at what expense to the environment and our health? Did our grandparents enjoy better health because they bottled summer produce for the winter and fermented veggies for later consumption? There is evidence that this is so.

Check labels and eat organic foods as much as possible. Why not grow your own and buy locally at farmers' markets?

Any politician or scientist that tells you that these (GMO) products are safe is either very stupid or lying.
> David Suzuki, scientist, geneticist, environmentalist

Genetically Engineered (GMO) varieties of corn, soya, sugar beets and canola have become common local crops in Canada. Apples, potatoes and wheat are all in the lineup for approval.

The safety to human consumption of genetically modified foods have not been proven and a growing body of research connects these foods with health concerns and environmental damage.

Besides the fact that such crops have never been adequately tested for safety, the EWG (Environmental Working Group) says that GMO foods are increasing the amount of herbicide-resistant weeds that no longer die when they are sprayed with Monsanto's Roundup, which the seeds were bred to resist.

From David Suzuki Foundation: http://www.davidsuzuki.org/ what-you-can-do/queen-of-green/faqs/food/understanding-gmo/

Glyphosate Drives Breast Cancer Proliferation, Study Warns, as Urine Tests Show Europeans have this Weed Killer in Their Bodies By Dr. Mercola

Disturbing discoveries relating to glyphosate — the active ingredient in Monsanto's broad-spectrum herbicide Roundup — keep emerging.

Now, testing shows that people in 18 countries across Europe have glyphosate in their bodies, while yet another study reveals that the chemical has estrogenic properties and drive breast cancer proliferation in the *parts-per-trillion* range. As reported by GreenMedinfo.com:

"Does this help explain the massive mammary tumors that the only long term animal feeding study on Roundup and GM corn ever performed recently found?"

Meanwhile, a new free trade agreement, known as the Transatlantic Trade and Investment Partnership (TTIP), has again cracked the door open for genetically engineered (GE) crops and foods into Europe.

This may effectively negate the hard work Europeans have done to limit the proliferation of genetically modified organisms (GMOs) in their food supply, and with genetically engineered "Roundup Ready" crops and the food made from it come increased glyphosate exposure...

People Across Europe Test Positive for Glyphosate

A 2011 study detected glyphosate in 60-100 percent of all US air and rain samples, and last year another study revealed widespread glyphosate contamination in groundwater. When groundwater is used as a drinking water source, this contamination poses a risk to animals, plants and humans alike.

Now, the first-ever test for weed killer contamination in human bodies was commissioned by Friends of the Earth Europe. Volunteers from 18 different countries provided urine samples.

Of the 182 urine samples tested, an average of 44 percent was found to contain glyphosate, although the proportion of contamination varied from country to country. All volunteers were city dwellers who had not handled or used glyphosate, and only one person per household was tested.

Macedonia and Bulgaria had the least number of positive tests (10 percent), while 90 percent of samples in Malta tested positive. Seventy percent of volunteers in Germany, UK and Poland had the weed killer in their bodies.

Can you even imagine what the results might be if similar testing was conducted in the US, considering the fact that Americans eat their own weight or more in genetically engineered foods each and every year—in large part because the US does not require GE foods to be labeled, so many are still completely in the dark about such stealth ingredients.

The fact that close to half of all people are testing positive for glyphosate (including countries that don't even use it) is profoundly disturbing in light of the recent findings that this commonly used weed killer may be among the most important factors in the development of modern diseases, as the pathway by which glyphosate kills plants is the identical pathway found in animal and human gut bacteria.

http://articles.mercola.com/sites/articles/archive/2013/06/25/glyphosate-residue.aspx

The PLU code, or price lookup number printed on the sticker on fruit, also tells you how the fruit was grown. By reading the PLU code, you can tell if the fruit was genetically modified, organically grown or produced with chemical fertilizers, fungicides, or herbicides.

A four-digit code beginning with a 3 or a 4 means the produce is probably conventionally grown. If there are five numbers in the PLU code, and the number starts with "9", this tells you that the produce was grown organically and is not genetically modified.

Someday we will look back on this dark era of agriculture and shake our heads in disbelief. How could we have ever believed it was a good idea to grow our food with poisons?

Jane Goodall

Prevention magazine reported: "There is increasing evidence that the dying of bees is linked to pesticides sprayed on crops. US regulations also prohibit organic dairy and livestock operations from using GMO grains (again, corn and soy) to feed their animals."

To learn more:
http://www.naturalnews.com/044332_GMOs_organic_food_ingredient_labeling.html#ixzz2wJsASfD3

- The European Union is considering banning the use of nicotinoids (insecticides) to treat seeds which have been related to the demise of bee colonies and also suspected of diminishing populations of wild birds who eat the seeds. Ontario is also phasing in restrictions of their use with an 80 per cent reduction in acreage planted with neonicotinoid-treated corn and soybean seed by 2017.

Powerhouse foods:
Garlic is anti-bacterial, anti-viral and anti-fungal, contains allicin, a chemical that is anti-carcinogenic as well as imparting many other health benefits. The key is to crush garlic and let it sit for 15 minutes in order to release these anti-cancer compounds. For optimal results, **garlic** should be fresh since the active ingredient is destroyed within one hour of smashing. Garlic from China is useless – it is irradiated for the long journey and comes to us devoid of taste and nutrients. Again, organic is best!

A double blind, randomized study with over 3000 human subjects for seven clinical years showed that cancer risk was cut by 60% for those with the highest intake of allium-containing vegetables (onions, garlic, chives, leeks, shallots and scallions) including aged garlic.

Flaxseeds are an excellent source of omega 3 fatty acids, fiber and lignans, components which support healthy immune function, provide antioxidant protection and fight inflammation.

University of Toronto researchers gave breast cancer patients muffins with 25 grams of ground flaxseeds. Another group of women were given muffins without flaxseeds. Both groups were awaiting treatment. Women who received the flaxseed muffins showed slower growing tumors but there was no change in the size or growth of the tumors in women who did not get the flaxseed muffins.

Spice things up! Add the cancer-fighters listed below. Many herbs and spices are concentrated sources of antioxidants. Fresh and dried herbs and spices also liven up your meals without sodium (that's good for your blood pressure) or extra calories.

Herbs and spices
- Turmeric
- Oregano
- Cinnamon
- Cloves: the highest of all foods tested

Oregano and **rosemary** are strong antioxidants. **Cilantro** seems to detoxify cancer-causing compounds. All are available as essential oils from doTerra.

Curcumin, the powerful yellow spice found in both **turmeric** and **curry** powders, has demonstrated major therapeutic potential in preventing breast cancer metastasis.

The antioxidant, anti-inflammatory and anti-carcinogenic properties of **curcumin** have been undergoing intense research in various parts of the world. **Curcumin** appears to be safe in the treatment of nearly all cancers, including multi-drug resistant cancers. In India, where the spice is widely used, the prevalence of the top four U.S. cancers – colon, breast, prostate and lung – is 10 times lower.

Extract of bitter melon may protect against breast cancer, researchers say. Eating bitter melon, rich in flavonoids and Vitamin C could also have beneficial effect.

Sulfur-containing vegetables such as broccoli, cabbage, cauliflower, kale and Brussels sprouts "turn off signals to cancer cells to divide and conquer."

Strawberries: The luscious red berries are rich in ellagic acid, a phytochemical that may function as an estrogen-blocker and thereby reduce hormone-driven breast cancers. At only 50 calories per cup, they're a cancer-fighter's friend as are anything that ends with "erry": raspberries, blueberries and cherries.

Pistachios: This green nut is full of gamma-tocopherol, a potentially cancer-fighting type of vitamin E. But that's not all: They're also rich in phytosterols, which give a double boost with its anti-cancer and heart-health properties. Plus, they provide a hefty amount of fiber and blood pressure-loving potassium.

The foods you eat have incredible power to heal -- or harm -- your body. Incorporate the following as much as you can into your daily diet:

> ➤ **Green tea:** Three cups of green tea a day can prevent breast cancer by as much as 50% because of its high antioxidant content. Squeezing a little lemon into your cup, can increase the antioxidant power 10 times. Besides being an excellent source of antioxidants, green tea is also packed with vitamins A, D, E, C, B, B5, H, and K, manganese, and other beneficial minerals such as zinc, chromium, and selenium.
> ➤ **Pomegranates** offer active and significant protection against breast cancer. They prevent estrogen and testosterone from rising too high in the body and block the stimulation of breast tissues with these hormones.
> ➤ **Seaweed, or** kelp, high in iodine, is a cancer-fighting agent, containing powerful anti-oxidants that inhibit the growth of certain cancer cells, mostly breast cancer. Crumble seaweed over salads, vegetables, soups and rice.
> ➤ In addition to **asparagus**'s many other nutritional benefits (low-calorie plus a good source of

vitamins, calcium, iron, thiamin, potassium and fiber), it is high in the micronutrient glutathione, an antioxidant. Glutathione is said to defend the body against viruses, certain types of cancer, and boosts immune cells.

A study of more than 2,000 Chinese women, found that the more fresh and dried **mushrooms** the women ate, the lower was their breast cancer risk. Women who consumed 4 grams or more of dried mushrooms were 50 per cent less likely to develop breast cancer than non-mushroom eaters. The risk was lower still among those who also drank green tea everyday.

Brazil nuts are an excellent source of organic **selenium**, a powerful antioxidant-boosting mineral that may help prevent cancer.

Eating the right foods is half the battle. How you cook it also affects your weight and cancer risk. Follow these healthy culinary tips:

> ➢ **Cook more meals at home.** You'll have more control over what you're putting into your body.
>
> **Do not char:** because of the high temperatures, grilling and frying meats, fish and poultry increases the formation of cancer-causing compounds.
>
> **Boiling vegetables** destroys or washes away some cancer-fighting nutrients. Instead, steam or bake in small amounts of liquid. For me, roasting with olive oil and herbs is the most flavourful.

Soy for Cancer Survivors?

Reports by several scientists in reputable publications and cancer foundations have stressed the importance of soy to reduce breast cancer. Meanwhile there has been plenty of research to contradict these claims and completely oppose them.

http://preventdisease.com/news/14/090714_Soy-Accelerates-Breast-Cancer-Rather-Than-Prevent-It.shtml

I'm not taking any chances and recommend you consider the following:

Researchers compared tumor tissues from before and after a 30-day regimen of consuming a soy supplement while a control group took a placebo. They found changes in the expressions of certain genes that are known to promote cell growth, in those women taking the soy supplement.

The findings led them to conclude the soy protein could potentially accelerate the progression of the disease and that soy may exert a stimulating effect on breast cancer in a sub set of women.

Any ingredient listed as soybean or soy on any product ingredient list has a 93% chance of being GMO if it is not listed as organic. But even organic soy cannot be trusted. Non-organic sources of soy in many agricultural practices are being passed off as organic.

Fermented sources of soy such as natto, miso, tempeh and some fermented tofu are likely the only types of soy that should be consumed by humans as long as they are non-GMO and organically grown.

Cancer-Boosters: Stay Away!

Just as certain foods ward off cancer, others can increase your risk. But you don't have to swear them off entirely – just limit how much you indulge in them. Here are a few of the American Institute for Cancer Research **http://www.aicr.org** (AICR)'s recommendations:

1. **Red meat:** Use meat as a side dish or condiment, not your plate's centerpiece. Eat no more than 18 ounces of cooked red meat – beef, pork and lamb – per week, or 2.5 ounces per day
2. **Processed meats:** Just savor them occasionally.
3. **Alcohol:** Although moderate drinking is linked with less heart disease, women have another worry. Even one drink per day poses a higher risk of breast cancer. A study of 185,000 postmenopausal women found that those who had 1-2 drinks per day were 32% more likely to develop hormone-sensitive breast cancer (the most common form) compared to non-drinkers, according to the National Institutes of Health and American Association of Retired Persons research. For women who had three or more drinks daily, the risk jumped to 51%. If you drink, limit to one standard drink per day for women and two for men.
4. **Sugar-sweetened drinks:** Avoid sugary drinks. Regular sodas and other high-calorie, low-nutrient foods make weight control harder and contribute to other unhealthy states.

Supplements

A study published in a medical journal showed that breast cancer survivors who take aspirin regularly may live longer and be less likely to see their cancer return. The study of more than 4,000 nurses showed that those who took aspirin – usually to prevent heart disease – had a 50% lower risk from dying from breast cancer and a 50% lower risk that the cancer would spread.

Compared to women who took no **aspirin,** those who took 2-5 aspirin per week were:

- 71% less likely to die from breast cancer
- 60% less like to develop metastatic breast cancer
- 47% less likely to die from any cause.

Among women living at least one year after a breast cancer diagnosis, aspirin use was associated with a decreased risk of distant recurrence and breast cancer death.

http://jco.ascopubs.org/content/28/9/1467.full.pdf+html?sid=51c5e653-ddfa-4b7d-b463-221f1a762ad0

Scientists have known for a long time that **Vitamin D** is important for calcium absorption and that there is a link between levels of D and diseases such as cancer and MS. A study published in *American Journal of Clinical Nutrition* found women taking **calcium and Vitamin** D showed 60% reduction in cancer risk.

Vitamin D is crucial for activating the immune system. Most is made by the body as a natural by-product of skin exposure to sunlight. It can also be found in fish liver oil, eggs and fatty fish such as salmon, herring and mackerel or taken as a supplement.

As people spend more and more time indoors (and use sunscreen) low levels of vitamin D are suffered, meaning T cells are poor at fighting infection. If T cells cannot find Vitamin D they fail to mobilize.

Researchers tracked 1455 patients in Shanghai for six years and found that those taking **ginseng** (Chinese have used ginseng for thousands of years to stay healthy and treat illness) were 30% less likely to die from cancer than non-users. Women who began taking 1.3 g of ginseng root per day after diagnosis reported more energy and better sleep. All had conventional cancer treatment.

Scientists reported in 2005 evidence that **Co-enzyme Q10** restored ability of cancer cells to kill themselves, while not impacting normal cells. **Coenzyme-Q10** production diminishes after age 40 and supplementing it is good for heart health as well. **Ubiquinol** is a converted form of CoQ-10 and is considered an anti-aging supplement.

Our toxic chemical exposure is nothing short of a calamity.
                                    Dr. David Suzuki, environmentalist

Chemical Exposure

Common household goods, personal care products, and even food and water, are major sources of chemical exposure that can lead to an accumulation of toxins in your body.

Endocrine disruptors (hormone-altering chemicals) are everywhere in our modern environment and causing much alteration to our internal chemical composition: increasing production of certain hormones; decreasing production of others; imitating hormones;

turning one hormone into another; interfering with hormone signaling; telling cells to die prematurely; competing with essential nutrients; binding to essential hormones; accumulating in organs that produce hormones.

The **keep-a-breast.org** and Environmental Working Group **ewg. org** websites feature 12 Hormone-Altering Chemicals and how to avoid them.

The 12 worst endocrine disruptors that you need to avoid are:

1. bpa
2. dioxin
3. atrazine
4. phthalates
5. perchlorate
6. fire retardants
7. lead
8. arsenic
9. mercury
10. per-fluorinated chemicals
11. organophosphate pesticides
12. glycol ethers

Personal Care Products

These toxins are everywhere, especially in the stash of bathroom personal care collection we accumulate. Toxic substances are found in sunscreens, soaps, shampoos, detergents and even toothpastes. **Sodium lauryl sulfate** is a common degreaser used in practically every soap, shampoo and toothpaste on the market today. The compound has been used in studies to induce mutation in bacteria and irritate skin. It has also shown to enter the heart, liver, lungs and brain from skin contact and has been proven to maintain residual levels once inside these organs.

Switch to organic and plant-based products to avoid the long-term toxic buildup caused by these dangerous chemicals. Prolonged toxicity is known to foster the development of cancer. Read your labels on all items purchased to improve your family's personal lives to assure there is no sodium laurel sulphate doing the opposite!

Gillian Deacon's book, *There's Lead in Your Lipstick: Toxins in Our Everyday Body Care and How to Avoid Them,* is a wonderfully written resource full of information and humour and good alternative suggestions.

It has been suggested that one of the main causes of breast cancer is the use of **antiperspirant**. Most products on the market are a combination of antiperspirant/deodorants. Again, look at the labels! Deodorant is fine; however **antiperspirant** can be very harmful because of the concentration of toxins that causes cell mutation.

The human body has few areas where it can eliminate toxins. Toxins are eliminated through perspiration. Antiperspirants, which contain aluminum, prevent you from perspiring, thereby inhibiting the body to eliminate toxins through the armpits. Women, who apply antiperspirant after shaving the underarms, increase the risk due to tiny injuries and skin irritations which allows harmful chemical components to penetrate more quickly into the body.

Natural News reports that two recent studies have linked aluminum to breast cancer. One study published in July 2013 found that breast cancer patients had significantly higher levels of aluminum in their nipple aspirate fluids when compared to a control group of healthy women without breast cancer. The study compared 19 breast cancer patients with 16 healthy women in a control group.

Another study published in the same journal found that aluminum can increase the spread of breast cancer cells. Because the malignancy or spread of cancer is correlated with increased mortality, this finding is highly significant.

Research continues to reinforce the need to avoid aluminum whenever possible. Limiting toxins such as aluminum in one's environment can reduce the likelihood of cancer **and** brain damage. Primary sources of aluminum include processed foods, personal care products and cosmetics, cookware and vaccines.

http://www.naturalnews.com/042235_aluminum_breast_cancer_environmental_toxins.html#ixzz2g60N7Bmc

What to avoid:

Foods that contain **aluminum** include processed cheese, table salt, baking powder, bleached flour, cake mixes, prepared dough and baby formula. Medicines that contain **aluminum** include antacids, buffered aspirin and painkillers.

You can make your own deodorant by mixing together:

> ¼ cup coconut oil
> ¼ cup baking soda
> ¼ cup arrow root powder

Store in refrigerator as the coconut oil tends to melt in summer heat.

The cosmetic and personal care product industries are unregulated for harmful ingredients and many contain aluminum powder, which the Environmental Working Group (EWG) lists as having high health concerns as a neurotoxin. Aluminum powder is found in 1,718 products listed in the EWG database. The personal care products based on toxicity of ingredients, found to contain toxic aluminum include:

- eye liner
- eye shadow
- mascara
- lip gloss
- nail polish
- hair spray
- deodorant
- dark hair color

Aluminum pans used for cooking have been shown to leach harmful aluminum into the food items that are cooked in them, so these should be eliminated whenever possible. Teflon is no better and ceramic-coated cookware is the new go-to safe non-stick cookware.

Almost all vaccines contain the heavy metal aluminum hydroxide in them, which is likewise considered to be a dangerous neurotoxin.

I remember reading in *Time* magazine, many years ago, that the fall of the Roman empire may have been due to lead poisoning because of the widespread use of lead: in aqueducts, makeup, and vessels for storing and drinking liquids. This caused impotency and also mental decline. Is this what we are unwittingly doing to our society today by using so many chemicals the impact of which we are unaware? Look at the increasing number of life-threatening allergies, early puberty, autism and the prevalence of auto-immune diseases and dementia, not to mention cancer!

Many people are now considering our increasingly polluted environment as a possible culprit in the increase in cancer cases. Breast cancer incidence in the North America has risen since World War II, when industry began pumping out pesticides, plastics, solvents, and other chemicals, leaving residues in our air, water, and soil. Laboratory studies suggest that many of these chemicals may cause breast tumors, hasten their growth, or leave mammary glands more vulnerable to carcinogens.

My grandmother, Carmela, was a wise and free-spirited, compassionate and loving woman. Born in Southern Italy, she kept up the heart-healthy Mediterranean diet during her forty years living in Canada. Indeed, if not for her hard-working life, she might have lived as long as her 98 year-old mother who died in Italy on her own organic olive and fruit farm. But that was not to be, for Nonna spent summers as crew boss picking the pesticide-laden fruits of Ontario's golden horseshoe. Sadly, she passed of cancer at a young 64. Her daughter, Maria Christina, my mother, has always been a health-conscious eater and, in 2015, is a healthy, vibrant, 94 year year-old!

Besides contributing to the pollution of the planet by using plastic water bottles, we are adding to our toxic load. One 2011 independent test revealed 38 contaminants in bottled water. Each of the 10 tested brands contained an average of eight chemicals. Disinfection byproducts (DBPs), caffeine, Tylenol, nitrate, industrial chemicals, arsenic, and bacteria were all detected.

Fluoride is also usually present in both tap water and filtered bottled water. Many health-conscious people search out spring water sources as a pure source for everyday consumption.

An Environmental Healer-Hero

Dr. Victor Cecilioni was known and respected internationally for his ground-breaking studies in the 1970s that showed cancer rates for people who lived near steel mills in industrialized cities were far higher than for those living elsewhere. He spent his lifetime crusading on behalf of factory workers in Ontario suffering from industrial disease and the North End Hamilton residents who struggled with industrial air pollution.

Dr. Victor also examined cancer death rates in various Canadian cities and found that the cancer death rate in areas with fluoridated water was 15-25% higher than areas with non-fluoridated water.

Fittingly, Environment Hamilton's annual **Environmentalist of the Year Award** named after him.

("*Caro Dottore*" as he was affectionately known by his Italian immigrant patients, is loved and respected by me for having brought me into this world and for treating my childhood illnesses — via many in-home visits — with this tender caring and thorough bedside manner. I wonder if he somehow unwittingly influenced my lifelong concern for the environment.)

For more information on fluoridation of drinking water visit: http://cof-cof.ca/

Hormone Replacement Therapy

North America saw a decline in breast cancer incidence in 2003 and 2004, a change that has been largely attributed to post-menopausal women discontinuing their **hormone replacement therapy** after research showed that it can cause breast cancer.

Taking menopause hormones for five years doubles the risk for breast cancer. Even women who took progesterone and estrogen pills for a couple of years had a greater risk of getting cancer. But the good news is that when they stopped taking the medication their odds quickly returned to normal roughly two years after quitting.

Ontario Breast Cancer Information Exchange Project publishes a pamphlet "Hormone Replacement Therapy for Breast Cancer Survivors" which outlines alternatives to HRT for menopausal women:

- For relief of hot flashes avoid alcohol and caffeine
- Wear layered clothing
- Increase intake of vitamin E
- A well balanced diet, low in fat and high in fibre is recommended for everyone
- Add flaxseed, soy, tofu and miso as excellent dietary sources of estrogen.
- Some common herbs to relieve symptoms include primrose oil, ginseng, Dong Quoi and black cohosh
- Exercise will keep bones and joints and heart healthy. Exercise will also help you sleep, digest food better, and increase your overall well-being.

Clothing

Clothes can affect our health as well; they come in close contact with our skin and emit particles that we breathe in.

Recommendations from Silent Spring Institute:

http://silentspring.org/your-selection-and-care-clothing

- **Choose clothing made from natural, untreated materials whenever possible.**
- **Avoid flame-retardant clothing, which has been treated with polybrominated diphenyl ethers, or PBDEs.**
- **Use dry cleaning services that do not use perchloroethylene (PERC) or request "wet cleaning."** If you must use traditional dry cleaning with PERC, open the plastic bag outdoors on a porch or in the garage, discard the plastic immediately, and air your clothes out before hanging them in a closet or wearing them.
- **Avoid commercial fabric softeners, which often contain undisclosed chemicals and harmful fragrances.**
- **Minimize your use of chlorine bleach.**
- **Avoid fluorescent whitening agents, also known as optical brighteners.**
- **Never use mothballs.**

Make your own fabric softener using baking soda or white vinegar. I use dryer balls. Norwex.ca has a couple of excellent choices which are environmentally friendly too: when using these balls you can reduce dryer time by 25 per cent. Even better, hang laundry to air dry using that old stand-by "solar energy"

Many physicians and researchers agree that wearing a tight-fitting bra can cut off lymph drainage, which may contribute to the development of breast cancer because your body will be less able to excrete all the toxins you're exposed to on a daily basis.

There are few solid studies on **bra wearing and breast cancer,** but one of the most compelling was completed by medical anthropologists Sydney Singer and Soma Grismaijer — authors of *Dressed to Kill: The Link Between Breast Cancer and Bras.* The study of over 4,000 women found that women who do not wear bras have a much lower risk of breast cancer: when comparing women who wore their bras 24 hours a day with those who did not wear bras at all, there was a 125-fold difference in risk. Based on the results of this study, the link between bras and breast cancer is about three times greater than the link between cigarette smoking and cancer.

Although this study did not control for other risk factors, which could have skewed their results, other studies have found similar compelling links. For example, a group of Japanese researchers found that wearing a girdle or bra can lower your levels of melatonin by 60 percent. The hormone melatonin is intimately involved with the regulation of your sleep cycles, and numerous studies have shown that melatonin has anti-cancer activities.

See more: www.http://organichealth.co/primary-causes-of-breast-cancer-youll-want-to-know/

A Breath of Fresh Air

In the late '80s, NASA and the Associated Landscape Contractors of America studied houseplants as a way to purify the air in space facilities. They found several plants that filter out common volatile organic compounds (VOCs). Plants can also help clean indoor air, which is typically far more polluted than outdoor air. Other studies have since been published in the *Journal of American Society of Horticultural Science*. The plants listed below, besides absorbing carbon dioxide and releasing oxygen as do all plants, eliminate significant amounts of benzene and remove other specific chemicals.

- Aloe Vera
- Spider plant
- Gerbera Daisy
- Snake plant (mother-in-law's tongue)
- Golden Pothos
- Cyrsanthemum
- Dracaena Marginata and Warnickii
- Ficus benjamina
- Chinese evergreen
- Bamboo palm
- Heart-leaf philodendron
- Peace lily

Cleaning product chemicals to avoid include 2-butoxyethanol, which the Environmental Protection Agency considers a human carcinogen and has been linked to cancer; alkylphenol ethoxylates, which can disrupt hormones; and ethanolamines, which can cause asthma. But because cleaning product companies aren't required to list most ingredients on their product labels it can be tough to know what to buy. However, Seventh Generation, an eco-friendly company, clearly lists their ingredients on their labels. A cleaning with a mixture of one part water and one part vinegar, or scrubbing surfaces with baking soda, both of which have natural antibacterial properties is a good, economical alternative.

I use Norwex (www.norwex.ca) microfiber cloths and am able to clean and sanitize with just plain water – no chemicals at all!

If you must use something other than water, try vinegar as your go-to, all-purpose cleaner. Acetic acid, or white vinegar, is a powerful natural disinfectant, safe for use on most surfaces. It also acts as a deodorizer, beats hard-water deposits, cuts grease and is completely biodegradable.

Breast Cancer Detection Methods

Finding a lump or mass in the breast is a sign of breast cancer, and you know it's important to seek immediate medical evaluation if a lump is detected. Fortunately, however, most breast lumps result from noncancerous conditions such as various types of cysts or injury, according to the Mayo Clinic.

And remember: Results from a Norwegian study of 200,000 women suggest that in 20% of cases, small cancerous changes and tumors in women's breasts may vanish without treatment.

Well, now, that you have done, one-step-at-a-time or all-embracing, what you can to avoid another bout with "Big C", you will maintain checkups with your health-care team and keep adding lifestyle improvements to keep it at bay. The following is some information about detection that you may find useful.

Mammography

Several studies over the past few years have concluded that mammograms do not save lives, and may actually harm more women than they help, courtesy of false positives, overtreatment, and radiation-induced cancers.

The latest study to reach this conclusion is also one of the longest and largest. As reported by the *New York Times*:

"One of the largest and most meticulous studies of mammography ever done, involving 90,000 women and lasting a quarter-century, has added powerful new doubts about the value of the screening test for women of any age.

It found that the death rates from breast cancer and from all causes were the same in women who got mammograms and those who did not. Besides that, the screening had damages: one in five cancers found with mammography and treated was not a threat to the woman's health and did not need treatment such as chemotherapy, surgery or radiation."

But then again...

Often-conflicting results from studies on the value of routine mammography serve to fuel the debate about how often women should get a mammogram and at what age they should start.

In a new analysis of previous research, experts re-examined the results of four large studies. All the studies showed a substantial reduction in breast cancer deaths with mammography screening.

Magnetic resonance imaging (MRI) is a diagnostic procedure that uses a combination of a large magnet, radio waves, and a computer to produce detailed images of organs and structures within the body.

MRI, used with mammography and breast ultrasound, can be a useful diagnostic tool. Recent research has found that MRI can locate some small breast lesions sometimes missed by mammography. It can also help detect breast cancer in women with breast implants and in younger women who tend to have dense breast tissue. Mammography may not be as effective in these cases. Since MRIs do not use radiation, they may be used to screen women younger than 40 and to increase the number of screenings per year for women at high risk for breast cancer.

Recent research has demonstrated that using commercially available software programs to enhance breast MRI scans can reduce the number of false positive results with malignant tumors, thereby reducing the need for biopsies.

Breast Thermography Health Assessment Imaging is a physiological test to monitor your breast health, allowing you the opportunity to address chronic inflammation in your body BEFORE cancer has had the time to develop.

Infrared cameras measure the heat coming from the surface of your body. Specialized software translates temperature data into thermal images for medical evaluation. It is non-invasive and does not utilize mechanical compression or ionizing radiation, and can alert us to physiological abnormalities due to inflammation or increased tumor-related blood flow, 8-10 years before mammography or a physical exam can detect a cancerous mass.

Breast Thermography Health Assessment Imaging benefits are proven effective for women of all ages and for all breast densities. It is particularly helpful for women with dense breasts, as they are at a higher risk of developing cancer, and have an increased risk of both false positives and false negatives due to the limitations mammograms have in imaging dense breast tissue.

Elastography

A new screening technique used in conjunction with ultrasound can reduce need for breast biopsies. New research finds **Elastography** which analyzes breast tumors increases diagnostic accuracy over ultrasound alone. Using this technique, scientists identified 98 per cent of malignant and 82 per cent deemed benign. Researchers see this technique as a way to eliminate needle biopsies for growths that are probably benign, giving definitive results earlier.

Future Diagnostic Techniques

➢ An anti-cancer vaccine tested on mice may be available for women within a decade.

New research suggests possible detection of cancer 17 months before a woman is diagnosed with the disease. Researchers found EFGR (epidermal growth factor receptor) **examining blood tests** given to 420 estrogen receptor-positive breast cancer patients before they were diagnosed. Blood tests were compared to blood from a control group. Those with the highest levels of the receptor were 2.9 times more likely to develop breast cancer than those with the least levels. **Identification of these proteins** could have a major impact on detecting breast cancer earlier when it is most treatable.

Physician and cancer researcher, Deborah Rhodes is an expert at managing breast-cancer risk. The director of the Mayo Clinic's Executive Health Program is now testing a **gamma camera** that can see tumors that get missed by mammography, uses one-fifth radiation dose — and is pain-free! Working with a team of physicists, Dr. Rhodes developed this new tool for tumor detection that is three times as effective as traditional mammograms for women with dense breast tissue.

In her Ted talk, https://wwww.ted.com/talks/deborah_rhodes# t-508168, Dr. Rhodes suggests:

- Know your breast density
- If premenopausal, book your mammogram for the first 2 weeks of your menstrual cycle when breast are less dense
- If you notice a persistent change insist on additional imaging

Hamilton, Ontario's McMaster University's CSii (Centre for Surgical and Scientific Innovation) is working with MDA, the creators of aerospace's Canadarm, to produce the first **Image Guided Automatic Robotic** (IGAR) system designed for early detection and treatment of breast cancer for high-risk patients.

Right now, high risk patients have MRI screenings, and IGAR could make those more accurate. It can be hard to pinpoint a mass during a separate biopsy, but when the biopsy is done while the patient is still in the MRI machine, it can be targeted more directly. Ideally, a mass could be detected, biopsied, and removed all in one visit. If a biopsy shows a tumor is very slow growing, then surgery can be avoided.

Dr. Mehran Anvari, Professor of Surgery, McMaster University, Hamilton, Ontario, and CEO and scientific director of CSii, predicts: "With this technology, if the MRI detects even the smallest lesion, the robot can actually go in and biopsy and we hope in future also potentially ablate the lesion."

There are other screening options, each with their own strengths and weaknesses, and you have a right to utilize those options. Also remember that in order to truly avoid breast cancer, you need to focus your attention on actual prevention and not just early detection.

Well quite a lot of information to digest? Making small changes — any changes —frequently and periodically, will give YOU more control. Once you decide to add certain foods to your everyday meals, to avoid certain chemicals and contaminants and add more physical activity, you will feel more empowered with each change. And having been successful incorporating these changes, you will be motivated to make even more adaptations.

But first, I urge you to see your place in the planet.

I was a small child playing on the kitchen floor with a small Stelco Credit Union savings bank. Embossed on the bank was a little cartoon man carrying an umbrella and his own credit union bank. The one he was carrying had embossed on it a little man carrying an umbrella and a bank which had embossed on it a little man carrying an umbrella ….. and so on and so on like an infinite Russian doll. I tried to imagine when it would end, this tiny image of a man carrying a bank. I realized there would be no ending no matter how small or how large the image I could see became. "That's how God is!"

The message hit me at age four and has never left. We are "as above so below", made in the image of God. Just like the man on the bank, we are intricately bound to all life in the universe. Life itself is a miracle as is the natural world around us. We need to awaken to spiritual beauty and the healing effects of nature. Studies repeatedly have shown that contact with nature can lower blood pressure, reduce anxiety, relieve stress, sharpen mental states and, among children with attention and conduct disorders, improve behavior and learning.

Many who have changed their way of life through expanded awareness find that their consciousness has made them more aware of other life forms and many begin living as they had never considered before. How many friends have become vegetarian either through compassion for the way animals are treated or for reasons of health and age-related disease prevention? As we learn more about the universe through the ever-increasing technological advances, we, in turn, expand our consciousness and what once fit no longer suits.

See your place on this planet. Our earth is the body of a Divine consciousness in which we live and breathe and have our being. Determine how you fit in and examine what you can do to help clean up the dis-ease that our earthly home is currently undergoing. It is up to us to "shrink the tumor" that threatens the home of future of generations.

As we promote healing in our physical bodies, we sow the seeds of healing of the Earth. What we do to rid our bodies of the toxicities of our environment enriches Earth and our expanding global consciousness promotes peace.

My most important advice is to be kind and loving to yourself. You are your own best friend and deserve the very best that life has to offer.

It is my prayer for you that you have a heart -and soul-enriching outcome, that you are healthier than ever before as a result of having traveled through "Cancer-Land" and that you continue the rest of your days, however many they may be, in heartfelt, life-affirming, resounding joy.

Namaste

Printed in the United States
By Bookmasters